Handbook of Diagnostic and Therapeutic Spine Procedures

Handbook of Diagnostic and Therapeutic Spine Procedures

Alan L. Williams, MD

Clinical Professor of Radiology
St. Louis University School of Medicine
St. Louis, Missouri

F. Reed Murtagh, MD

Professor of Radiology, Neurology, and Neurosurgery
Director, Neuroradiology
University Diagnostic Institute
University of South Florida
Tampa, Florida

Victoria, CMI

Medical Illustrator

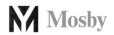 Mosby

An Imprint of Elsevier Science

St. Louis   London   Philadelphia   Sydney   Toronto

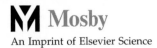

Mosby

An Imprint of Elsevier Science

11830 Westline Industrial Drive
St. Louis, Missouri 63146

Notice

Medicine is an ever-changing field. Standard safety precautions must be followed, but as
new research and clinical experience broaden our knowledge, changes in treatment and
drug therapy may become necessary or appropriate. Readers are advised to check the
most current product information provided by the manufacturer of each drug to be
administered to verify the recommended dose, the method and duration of administration,
and contraindications. It is the responsibility of the treating physician, relying on experience and knowledge of the patient, to determine dosages and the best treatment for each
individual patient. Neither the Publisher nor the Editor assumes any liability for any
injury and/or damage to persons or property arising from this publication.

The Publisher

Acquisitions Editor: Stephanie Donley
Production Editor: Edna Dick
Production Manager: Guy Barber
Illustration Specialist: Robert Quinn

Printed in the United States of America

International Standard Book Number 0323017177

Last digit is the print number: 9 8 7 6 5 4 3 2 1

To our wives, Luanne and Dorrie,
And our children, Allison, Gregory and Lindsay; Ryan and Kevin
They bring great joy to our lives.

A.L.W.
F.R.M.

Contributors

Farshad M. Ahadian, MD, Assistant Clinical Professor of Anesthesiology, University of California, San Diego, School of Medicine; Center for Pain and Palliative Medicine, University of California, San Diego, Medical Center, La Jolla, California
Pulsed Radiofrequency Techniques in Clinical Practice

Thomas D. Berg, MD, Clinical Lecturer, Department of Radiology, University of Iowa Hospitals and Clinics; Partner, Radiologic Medical Services, P.C., Mercy Hospital, Iowa City, Iowa
Epidurography and Epidural Steroid Injections

Leo F. Czervionke, MD, Associate Professor, Department of Radiology, Mayo Medical School, Rochester, Minnesota; Consultant, Mayo Clinic, Jacksonville, Florida
Discography

Robert H. Dorwart, MD, Center for Diagnostic Imaging, Indianapolis, Indiana
Spinal Facet and Sacroiliac Joint Blocks

Timothy S. Eckel, MD, MS, Part-time Assistant Professor of Neuroradiology (Teaching Affiliation), Johns Hopkins Medical Institutions, Baltimore; Director of Neuroradiology, Anne Arundel Medical Center and Annapolis Radiology Associates, Annapolis, Maryland
Intradiscal Electrothermal Therapy

Georges Y. El-Khoury, MD, Professor of Radiology, Department of Radiology, University of Iowa Hospitals and Clinics, Iowa City, Iowa
Epidurography and Epidural Steroid Injections

Douglas S. Fenton, MD, Assistant Professor, Department of Radiology, Mayo Medical School, Rochester, Minnesota; Consultant, Mayo Clinic, Jacksonville, Florida
Discography

Glen K. Geremia, MD, Professor, Departments of Radiology and Neurosurgery, Rush-Presbyterian-St. Luke's Medical Center, Chicago, Illinois
Percutaneous Needle Biopsy of the Spine

Wendell A. Gibby, MD, Director of MRI, Utah Valley Regional Medical Center, Provo, Utah
Automated Percutaneous Lumbar Discectomy

John M. Mathis, MD, MSc, Clinical Associate Professor of Radiology, University of Pennsylvania School of Medicine, Philadelphia, Pennsylvania; Chairman, Department of Radiology, Lewis-Gale Medical Center, Roanoke, Virginia
Percutaneous Vertebroplasty

F. Reed Murtagh, MD, Professor of Radiology, Neurology, and Neurosurgery, Director, Neuroradiology, University of South Florida, University Diagnostic Institute, Tampa, Florida
Intraspinal Cyst Aspiration

Andrew L. Wagner, MD, Director of Neuroradiology, Department of Radiology, Ruckingham Memorial Hospital, Harrisonburg, Virginia
Intraspinal Cyst Aspiration

Alan L. Williams, MD, MBA, Clinical Professor of Radiology, St. Louis University School of Medicine, St. Louis, Missouri
Myelography

Wade Wong, DO, Professor of Radiology, Department of Radiology, University of California, San Diego, Medical Center/Thornton Hospital, La Jolla, California
Spinal Nerve Blocks

Foreword

Neuroradiology began as a purely diagnostic specialty of radiology, identifying and localizing diseases of the brain and the spine. The first stirrings of further specialization appeared in the early 1970s with the birth of interventional neuroradiology, a field requiring such detailed expert skill and knowledge that it necessitated the concentrated attention of the practitioner.

The introduction of computed tomography (CT), also in the first half of the 1970s, produced an order-of-magnitude increase in the information obtained imaging the brain, otolaryngologic areas, and the spine. Once again many neuroradiologists realized that concentration of their efforts in one anatomic area was necessary to understand all of the anatomic, physiologic, and pathologic information that had become available. One of the neuroradiologists who dedicated his primary efforts to the spine was Alan L. Williams. His work and his publications, with Victor M. Haughton and others, in both spine CT and in magnetic resonance imaging (MRI) of the spine, have elucidated imaging anatomy and disease processes and have helped establish the intellectual basis for interventional spine procedures.

In the meantime, interventional neuroradiology evolved into a full-time subspecialty of neuroradiology, employing minimally invasive techniques to contribute to the well-being of many patients. However, the dynamic practitioners of this field have chosen to limit their horizon to the vascular system, showing no interest in the treatment of diseases of the spine. So, while anesthesiologists, neurologists, and other clinicians have become "spine pain physicians," radiologists, until very recently, have stood aloof. A search for "facet and block" in the title/abstract database of the journal *Radiology* from 1965 to the present found only 4 publications, none since 1984!

There was one major, active, noisy exception to the absence of radiologists in spine intervention, and that was F. Reed Murtagh, who for many years has been the "voice in the wilderness," telling radiologists that they should be doing these procedures because they can do them best; telling them that radiologists are uniquely qualified by selection and training in the use of imaging for precise needle placement. With Reed beating the drum, the American Society of Spine Radiology for their 3rd annual symposium added "Image-Guided Interventions" as a major part of the program. The response was overwhelming and has remained so.

Now radiologists' titles are changing to become "spine interventionalists" or "spine interventional neuroradiologists," and it is good to see radiology expanding into new territory rather than clinical specialties encroaching on radiology. And we *can* do it better!

Now Alan Williams and Reed Murtagh have produced this *Handbook for Diagnostic and Therapeutic Spine Procedures*, the first textbook by radiologists describing minimally invasive spine techniques. This is a book that guides the reader in detail through the use of imaging to accomplish each procedure. It is so comprehensive that it is more properly termed an "encyclopedia" than a "handbook." I have been privileged to review a number of chapters and have found them to be so well done, detailed, and clear that, having never done a facet block or epidural injection, I foolishly felt confident that I could go out and do one (but resisted the temptation). Different authors wrote each chapter, but the diligence of the editors has ensured that they are all equally detailed, with sufficient excellent figures. Each chapter follows the same format to such an extent that they could all have been written by the same person.

My thanks to Drs. Williams and Murtagh for giving me the opportunity to write this foreword. Congratulations to them for producing this needed seminal textbook, one that I believe will be a required, prized possession of all neuroradiologists, radiologists, and clinicians with an interest in minimally invasive spine procedures.

IRVIN I. KRICHEFF, MD
Emeritus Professor and Research Professor of Radiology,
New York University School of Medicine

Preface

This book is designed as a handy reference guide for those physicians performing diagnostic and/or therapeutic procedures related to the spine. These procedures have been requested by referring physicians with increasing frequency in recent years and currently represent an important segment of the diagnostic and therapeutic armamentarium for spine disease. The book is intended primarily for the radiologist in clinical practice who is getting started with these procedures as well as for fellows and residents.

Each chapter describes a specific diagnostic or therapeutic spine procedure and is contributed by one or more physicians who have had extensive clinical experience with the procedure. All chapters are organized in the same format, with the procedure described in a detailed, step-by-step presentation. Each technique is discussed in terms of rationale, clinical indications, contraindications, informed consent, pertinent anatomy, equipment and supplies, sedation, the actual procedure steps, post-procedure care, reporting, current coding, and a list of readings. This book is not designed to be a comprehensive description of spinal anatomy or pathology, but we hope that the detailed format and illustrations will be helpful in developing the appropriate clinical and technical expertise. More detailed anatomy and pathology may be obtained from numerous available textbooks.

We hope readers will find this handbook useful and informative as they seek to incorporate these techniques into their daily clinical practices.

ALAN L. WILLIAMS
F. REED MURTAGH

Acknowledgments

Many individuals have contributed to the reality of this project. We wish to thank each of the contributing authors for their timely and authoritative chapters. This volume is truly state-of-the-art because of their efforts. Thanks to Lois Hebel, Joann Shipp, and Louise Marshall at St. Louis University for their assistance in manuscript preparation. We greatly appreciate the effort and professionalism of the staff at Harcourt Health Sciences, especially Beth Staples, Victoria Heim, Guy Barber, Sally Grande, and Edna Dick. Special thanks to Stephanie Donley for her unrelenting encouragement and assistance during this project. David L. Daniels, MD and Leighton P. Mark, MD provided valuable suggestions for fine-tuning portions of the manuscript.

Additional thanks extended to Irvin I. Kricheff, MD, who has long been recognized as one of the most highly regarded academic neuroradiologists in the world. He has played a major role in the historical development of the subspecialty of neuroradiology. At New York University Dr. Irvin Kricheff nurtured more neuroradiology fellows and academic staff than he would probably care to admit. Although neither one of us has had the good fortune to work directly with Irv, he has been extremely supportive of our own careers. We are grateful for his mentoring and continued friendship and thank him for his willingness to contribute the Foreword for this book.

Contents

9

10

11

1

Epidurography and Epidural Steroid Injections

Thomas D. Berg, M.D.
and Georges Y. El-Khoury, M.D.

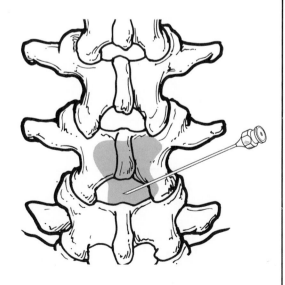

I.   Rationale for Procedure and Clinical Indications for Epidural Steroid Injections

A. Epidural steroid injection is a commonly requested procedure for the relief of upper and lower back pain due to:

  1. Spinal stenosis

  2. Disc herniation with or without sciatica

  3. Refractory back pain of uncertain etiology

B. Epidural steroid injections can help delay or possibly avoid surgical intervention. Many patients receive significant pain relief from epidural steroid injections that allows them to endure the acute pain flare and return to their usual activities with conservative management. The treatment process, however, may require more than one injection.

C. Epidural steroid injections combined with a dedicated regimen of anti-inflammatory medications and physical therapy can help provide satisfactory primary pain relief in patients who are not surgical candidates. (Epidural steroid injections have been used by anesthesiologists for pain relief since 1901.)

D. The ability of epidural steroids to alleviate pain of spinal origin was first described by Sicard in the early 1900s. Since that time there have been multiple investigations into the efficacy and mechanism of action of epidural steroids. The majority of these reports have stated that the proposed mechanism is a decrease in nerve root inflammation and swelling at the nerve-disc interface. Other authors have hypothesized that fluid alone injected into the epidural space interposes itself between the nerve root and disc, thereby mechanically influencing the pressure effect on the nerve root. Finally, some authors have stated that injections of steroid, with the addition of an anesthetic, may break a "pain cycle" and allow the patient to begin to recover from the initial insult. Regardless of the method of action, epidural steroid injections are efficacious in many patients, and they continue to function as front-line therapy for several back pain conditions.

II.   Contraindications

A. Absolute: Anticoagulation. Patients being treated with warfarin (coumadin) should discontinue treatment for 5 days; anticoagulation parameters (prothrombin time [PT], partial thromboplastin time [PTT], and international normalized ratio [INR]) should be rechecked prior to performing the injection. Aspirin is not an absolute contraindication; however, antiplatelet medications such as Plavix should be discontinued. Discussion of the risks and benefits with the referring physician is recommended on a case-by-case basis.

B. Relative: Allergy to contrast medium. In patients who are allergic to radiographic contrast medium, injections can be safely performed utilizing the loss of resistance technique with a cervical or lumbar approach, thereby eliminating the need to perform epidurography in this limited instance. Of course radiographic confirmation of needle placement is forgone.

III. Informed Consent

A. All patients are informed of the risks and benefits of the procedure and informed consent is obtained.

B. Potential risks associated with the lumbar or caudal approaches include hemorrhage, infection, vessel or nerve root injury, arachnoiditis, headache, contrast reaction, hypotensive response, and vasovagal episode. We have successfully utilized the sacral approach since 1983, with thousands of injections resulting in only a single infection, no cases of hemorrhage, no instances of vessel or nerve root injury, and no reported arachnoiditis or contrast reaction. The most common complication appears to be the vasovagal episode, which occurs in a percentage of cases similar to that of other needle-based procedures performed in other areas of the body. We have had two hypotensive episodes with the addition of Marcaine with epidural steroid. We no longer perform this injection at our institution due to the increased risks and monitoring necessary with anesthetic injections (described in detail in section VII). Headache risk is lower than that seen with myelograms and is directly proportional to the number of wet taps (a puncture that enters the subarachnoid space) that occur with the lumbar or cervical interlaminar approach.

C. Cervical steroid injections encompass the previously noted risks, with the additional risk of spinal cord injury. The possibility of spinal cord or nerve root injury should be discussed in depth with the patient so that there is absolute cooperation during the procedure. Additional emphasis should be placed on the possibility of hemorrhage in the cervical spine, because the secondary ramifications (spinal cord compression) are more serious than the potential problems associated with the lumbar or caudal approach. We routinely mention the possible need for emergency decompression surgery in the informed consent form because the patient must be fully aware of the risks and potential complications of the procedure. Performance of fluoroscopic visualization and cervical epidurography may decrease the risk of spinal cord injury by ensuring accuracy of needle placement.

IV. Pertinent Anatomy

A. Epidural space: The epidural space is a potential space that extends from the foramen magnum to the sacral hiatus (Fig. 1–1). The space is

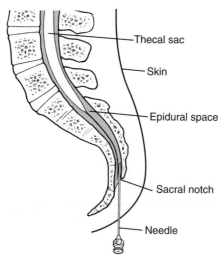

Figure 1-1. The epidural space is a potential space that extends from the foramen magnum to the sacral hiatus. Correct placement of the needle into the canal is shown.

located between the ligamentum flavum and the thecal sac. The epidural space contains the nerve roots and their dural investment, adipose tissue, veins, and loose areolar tissue. A midline septum (the plicae mediana dorsalis) can be observed in the sacral level. Although usually partial, this septum can rarely separate the sacral epidural space into right and left compartments.

B. Sacral approach

1. Sacral hiatus: The opening to the sacral hiatus can be palpated as a bony ridge normally located at the superior aspect of the natal cleft. The needle is advanced into the canal with a twisting motion to avoid its lodging in the periosteum or the bone itself. Correct placement is shown in lateral view in Figure 1–1. Note that it is important to superimpose the patient's hips in the lateral position so that rotation is eliminated.

2. Care should be exercised with osteoporotic patients, as their bone is soft and the needle can be advanced through the sacrum into the perirectal tissues.

3. Sacral epidurogram: The needle position is checked via injection of approximately 5 ml of low osmolar contrast (Omnipaque 180) to outline the epidural space and nerve roots. A normal AP epidurogram, shown in Figure 1–2, demonstrates contrast outlining the nerve roots and flowing freely from the needle.

   a. Care is taken to ensure that the needle is not placed in an epidural vein. This is done by checking for contrast medium flowing away

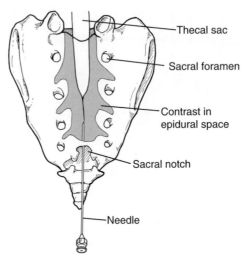

Figure 1–2. Normal AP epidurogram demonstrating contrast medium outlining the nerve roots and flowing freely from the needle.

in a cephalad direction in a vessel. The needle must be repositioned (usually anteriorly in the canal because the venous plexus lies posteriorly) until contrast is present only in the canal.

  b. The epidurogram is also inspected to confirm extradural position of the needle.

C. Lumbar approach

  1. Epidural space: Lies between the dural sac, ligamentum flavum, and vertebral bones. Figure 1–3 demonstrates the needle resting on the lamina adjacent to the interlaminar space.

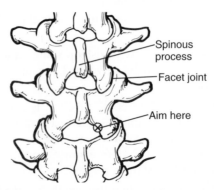

Figure 1–3. Indicates correct placement of the needle on the lamina adjacent to the interlaminar space.

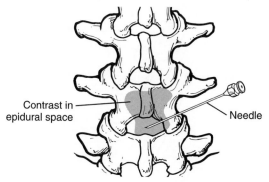

Figure 1–4. Loss of resistance technique is used to determine needle placement within the epidural space.

2. The needle is then "walked off" the lamina medially. Once by the lamina, the needle is slowly advanced using the loss of resistance technique (watching contrast for rapid forward motion as the column is "bounced"). Bouncing the contrast column refers to rapid tapping of the plunger of the medallion syringe as the Tuohy needle is slowly advanced. When the needle reaches the epidural space, the contrast column will rush toward the needle tip, and the needle is advanced no farther. Epidurography is then performed to confirm epidural placement (Fig. 1–4).

D. Cervical approach

Interlaminar approach at C7-T1 (Fig. 1–5). The needle is checked in the lateral position to ensure that it has not been advanced distal to the spinolaminar line (Fig. 1–6A). Once the lamina has been reached, the needle is "walked off" in a medial direction and slowly advanced while the contrast column is "bounced." The contrast rushes forward toward the needle tip as the epidural space is entered (Fig. 1–6B). AP cervical approach with cervical epidurogram is shown in Figure 1–7.

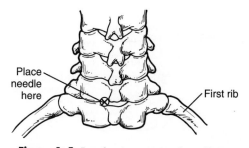

Figure 1–5. Interlaminar approach at C7-T1.

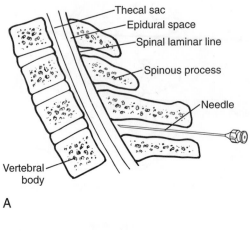

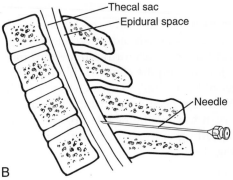

Figure 1-6. *A,* The needle is checked in the lateral position to ensure that it has not been advanced distal to the spinolaminar line. *B,* Once the lamina has been reached, the needle is "walked off" in a medial direction and slowly advanced while the contrast column is "bounced." The contrast agent rushes forward toward the needle tip as the epidural space is entered.

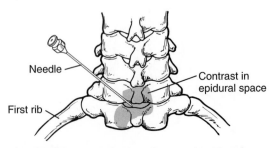

Figure 1-7. AP approach with cervical epidurogram.

V. Equipment Requirements

A. Epidural tray, all approaches

1. 3 ml Celestone Soluspan 6 mg/ml purchased in 5 ml vials. Agitate before injection. We use Celestone exclusively for joint and spine applications.

2. K50 connector tubing (20 cm)

3. 1% lidocaine, buffered with sodium bicarbonate

4. Syringes

   a. (3) 6 ml for local anesthetic, Celestone, and preservative-free saline (sacral approach)

   b. (1) 20 ml syringe for contrast (substitute a Medallion syringe for lumbar and cervical approach)

5. Omnipaque 180 or other low osmolar contrast agent such as Isovue

6. Sterile gauze pads (4 × 4's)

7. Betadine and alcohol for sterile scrub

8. Sterile towels or plastic fenestrated drape

B. Additional requirements for tray

1. Sacral approach: 22-gauge spinal needle, 3 ml preservative-free saline. The saline is used to advance the injected Celestone farther cephalad from the sacral approach. It is important to use preservative-free saline, since normal saline can cause precipitate formation when mixed with Celestone.

2. Lumbar approach: 22-gauge Tuohy needle with a Medallion syringe. Medallion syringes are more expensive; however, they provide improved tactile sensation and are essential for the lumbar and cervical approaches. Some radiologists advocate usage of a pillow under the abdomen to splay the spinous processes and open the interlaminar space as well.

3. Cervical approach: 22-gauge Tuohy needle with a Medallion syringe. A pillow or rolled towel is used to flex the patient's neck during the procedure.

C. Fluoroscopy unit

1. Epidurography and epidural steroid injections are most easily performed with access to dedicated C-arm equipment.

2. The sacral approach can be performed with a standard fluoroscopic table unit if the patient is able to assume the left lateral decubitus position.

3. The lumbar epidural steroid injection can be performed with a standard fluoroscopic unit with the patient remaining in the prone position throughout the entire procedure.

4. A dedicated C-arm is recommended for the cervical epidural approach to more easily define the pertinent anatomy and localize needle placement without requiring the patient to move. Patient movement increases the risk of nerve or cord injury.

D. Surgical gloves

1. Powder should be wiped from the gloves using alcohol or sterile saline. Powder is a potential source for adhesive arachnoiditis.

2. We use powder-free gloves for all procedures.

3. Always screen patients for latex allergies.

VI.   Sedation

A. No conscious sedation is required for the procedure. Detailed discussion of the procedure with emphasis on its brief duration will help calm the overly anxious patient, and the procedure can then be performed in the usual manner without the need for sedation. The patient's blood pressure is obtained prior to and following the procedure.

B. The extremely anxious patient may request conscious sedation. This may be deemed appropriate after review of the case.

1. Conscious sedation should proceed in accordance with each institution's policies.

2. Our facility generally utilizes a Versed and fentanyl regimen.

a. Midazolam (Versed): 0.5–1.5 mg IV administered over 2 minutes. Respiratory depression can occur in elderly patients.

b. Fentanyl can be used for pain relief at a dose of 25 μg with titration upward in accordance with the patient's body weight, age, and qualitative sensation of pain.

3. Continuous monitoring of the patient with pulse oximetry by a nurse is mandatory if conscious sedation is to be utilized. The nurse monitors the respiratory status, blood pressure, oxygen saturation, and heart rate. Values are recorded in the patient's chart.

4. Access to drugs such as flumazenil (Romazicon), a benzodiazepine-receptor antagonist, should be readily available to reverse the sedation, should the need for this arise.

5. Patients having conscious sedation must undergo a supervised recovery period for a minimum of 30–60 minutes following the final dose. This substantially increases the cost and time of procedure and decreases throughput (number of cases able to be treated in a given period of time) capabilities, while straining often limited nursing resources. Therefore, conscious sedation is provided only in extreme circumstances at our institution.

C. Uncooperative or agitated patients are not candidates for epidural steroid injection.

VII.   Procedure

A. Blood pressure: The patient's blood pressure is obtained prior to the procedure and recorded in the patient record.

B. All imaging studies pertinent to the procedure (cervical or lumbar spine magnetic resonance imaging [MRI], cervical or lumbar spine plain films) are reviewed prior to performing the procedure.

    1. Special attention is directed to the level of the thecal sac in the sacrum for sacral approach, the C7-T1 level for the cervical approach, and the size of the interlaminar spaces in the cervical and lumbar approaches.

    2. The levels of disc abnormalities, the conus, and any unusual findings are also reviewed prior to performing the injection.

    3. Stenotic levels, herniated discs, and so on should be avoided. The sacral approach is often preferred for elderly patients for this reason.

    4. The lumbar epidural injection is most efficacious at or one level below the most significant spinal stenosis or neural foramina narrowing.

C. Caudal approach: The patient is placed in the prone position and the sacral hiatus is palpated and the skin marked. Alternatively, the patient can be rolled into the left lateral decubitus position (standard fluoroscopic unit) and the sacral hiatus marked under fluoroscopic visualization.

    1. With the patient in the prone position, a small gauze pad is placed below the level of the puncture (outside the sterile field) between the buttocks in an attempt to absorb any betadine and/or alcohol that drips toward the perineal region. This can be very irritating to this sensitive skin region and uncomfortable for the patient. Aseptic technique with thorough scrubbing with sterile 4 × 4 pads soaked in betadine is essential to avoid an intraspinal infection. The betadine should be allowed to dry on the surface to maximize its antibacterial effect. The area is then wiped with alcohol, and a fenestrated drape is placed over the field.

    2. Approximately 1–2 ml of 1% buffered lidocaine is administered with a 25-gauge needle for a skin wheal for subcutaneous anesthesia of the sacral region. The needle is then advanced in the direction of the puncture to the level of the periosteum and 1–2 ml of 1% lidocaine is again administered for additional anesthesia. Buffering is performed with the addition of 5 ml of sodium bicarbonate to the 1% lidocaine vial. This raises the pH of the solution and results

in less burning sensation for the patient. The vial is used only once and then disposed of to reduce the chance of infection.

3. A 22-gauge needle is inserted into the epidural space at an angle of 45 degrees or less with a twisting motion in an attempt to advance the needle without lodging it in the periosteum.

4. The needle position is confirmed in the left lateral decubitus position (use of a C-arm obviates the need for the left lateral decubitus position). It is important to check the hips during fluoroscopy to confirm that they overlap and that there is no rotation present. If the needle is positioned superficial to the canal, the needle can be withdrawn and reinserted at the level of the hiatus under direct fluoroscopic visualization. Note that the actual advancement of the needle into the canal is easier in the prone position.

5. The needle should not be advanced farther than the S2 level due to the risk of entering the subarachnoid space above this level.

6. Once the needle is in the correct location, the stylet is removed and the patient is asked to perform a Valsalva maneuver to check for cerebrospinal fluid leakage.

7. The patient is again placed in the prone position and approximately 3 ml of Omnipaque 180 is injected to confirm epidural position of the needle and exclude positioning within an epidural vein. If epidural veins are visualized, the needle is readjusted until contrast medium is seen to remain within the epidural space. Note that the epidural venous plexus lies posteriorly, so that every attempt is made to move the needle more anterior in the canal.

8. If the patient complains of significant pain during the attempted injection and contrast simply pools in one spot, the needle is likely within the bone. The needle can be withdrawn slightly and reinjection attempted. If there is continued pain, the lateral position should be checked and the needle may have to be reinserted.

9. If the contrast fills the subarachnoid space, the procedure should be canceled and rescheduled for one week later.

10. A spot film is acquired to document positioning.

11. 3 ml of Celestone and 3 ml of preservative-free saline are then injected into the epidural space and the needle removed. During the injection, the patient may perceive temporary pain or a dull ache down the lower extremity. These symptoms usually abate if the injection is slowed or stopped.

12. Patients with acute back pain can be injected with 5–10 ml of 0.25% Marcaine as indicated. If Marcaine is administered during the injection, the patient must undergo a dedicated recovery with nurse supervision. The patient remains on a cart, and heart rate,

neurovascular status, pulse, and respiratory rate should be monitored every 15 minutes for at least 45 minutes. If the vital signs are stable, the patient's head can be raised to 45 degrees. The head is elevated gradually until the patient can tolerate the 90-degree upright position without dizziness or nausea. The patient must void and ambulate prior to physician examination and discharge.

13. The patient's blood pressure is obtained following the procedure and home care instructions are provided to the patient, warning of signs of infection and other complications. The patient then signs a release form, which includes the phone number for the radiology department and that of a 24-hour pager in case of a complication. A copy of the form is placed in the chart and the patient is released.

D. Complications: Complications in the sacral approach include misplacing the needle into the soft tissues or into or through the sacrum in osteoporotic patients. The needle could also traverse the thecal sac. Hemorrhage, infection, and contrast medium reaction are additional complications.

E. Lumbar approach: Utilizing fluoroscopic visualization, the lumbar level is checked and the interlaminar space is marked with a felt-tip marker such as a Sharpie.

1. The area is prepped with sterile 4 × 4 pads soaked with betadine. The betadine should be allowed to dry on the surface to maximize its antibacterial effect. The area is then wiped with alcohol. A fenestrated drape is then placed over the field in such a manner that a second level can be attempted without a second prep if this becomes necessary.

2. Approximately 3–5 ml of 1% buffered lidocaine is administered with a 25-gauge needle for subcutaneous anesthesia. Buffering is performed with addition of 5 ml of sodium bicarbonate to the vial of 1% lidocaine. This raises the pH of the solution and causes less burning sensation for the patient. The solution is used once and then discarded to reduce the chance of infection.

3. Using fluoroscopic visualization, a 22-gauge Tuohy needle is advanced to the level of the lamina. Once the needle is on the periosteum, it is carefully "walked off." This is accomplished by withdrawing the needle a couple of millimeters and then advancing it medially to slide past the lamina. The needle is advanced only as far as necessary to bypass the lamina.

4. Once the needle is past the lamina, the stylet is removed and a Medallion syringe with short (20 cm) K50 connecting tubing containing Omnipaque 180 is connected to the needle. The needle is then advanced while the contrast column is rapidly "bounced" (described in section IV. C.). Epidural placement is confirmed when the

contrast column rapidly advances toward the needle owing to loss of resistance in the epidural space. Visual inspection of the needle with stylet removed is also performed to ensure extradural position.

5. Approximately 3 ml of Omnipaque 180 is then injected into the epidural space for confirmation of correct positioning. The injection should outline the epidural nerve roots and flow freely from the needle. If only a single nerve root is seen, the needle should be adjusted and reinjection performed to ensure free flow of contrast medium in the epidural space.

6. A spot film is acquired to document positioning; this is essential for medicolegal purposes.

7. 3 ml of Celestone is then injected directly into the epidural space and the needle removed.

8. The patient is given a form warning of potential complications to watch for along with the phone number of the radiology department and that of a 24-hour pager in case of complications. The patient signs the form and a copy is placed in the medical record.

F. Complications of the lumbar approach include bleeding, infection, placement of needle into the subarachnoid space, and contrast medium reaction.

G. Cervical approach: The patient is placed into prone position with a pillow under the neck, which is flexed slightly forward in order to splay the spinous processes and widen the interlaminar space.

1. The C7-T1 spinous processes are palpated and the correct level is checked under fluoroscopic visualization. The skin is marked with a Sharpie marker.

2. The skin is prepped with sterile 4 × 4 pads soaked in betadine, and a fenestrated drape is placed over the field.

3. Approximately 5 ml of buffered 1% lidocaine is injected for subcutaneous anesthesia.

4. A 22-gauge Tuohy needle is then inserted under fluoroscopic visualization to the level of the lamina. The lateral fluoroscopic position is checked to confirm the needle is proximal to the spinolaminar line.

5. The Medallion syringe with short (20 cm) K50 connector tubing filled with Omnipaque 180 is then attached to the needle. Longer tubing reduces tactile sensation and makes the procedure more cumbersome.

6. The needle is advanced medially into the interlaminar region slowly while the contrast column is rapidly bounced, checking for loss of resistance, which signifies position in the epidural space. The distance to the epidural space is noticeably shorter with this approach

than with the lumbar approach; therefore, extreme care is used when advancing the needle.

7. Position is confirmed by injection of approximately 3 ml of Omnipaque 180 within the epidural space. The contrast medium should flow freely from the needle and outline the epidural nerve roots.

8. A spot film is obtained to document epidural positioning. This is very important medicolegally.

9. 3 ml of Celestone is then administered through the needle and the needle removed.

10. The patient is given a form listing potential complications and contact phone number for the department of radiology, and a 24-hour pager number in case of complications. The patient signs the form and a copy is placed in the medical record.

G. Complications of the cervical approach are identical to those with the lumbar approach, with the additional risk of cord injury.

VIII. Post-procedure Care

A. Following the procedure, the patient's blood pressure is recorded.

B. Care should be taken when the patient leaves the supine position to avoid a vasovagal reaction with subsequent fall from the fluoroscopy table. In our experience, athletes and young males seem to be particularly susceptible to this complication. If the patient experiences a vasovagal reaction, his or her feet should be immediately elevated and the table placed in Trendelenburg position to augment venous return and blood flow to the brain. Blood pressure, pulse oxygenation, lung sounds, and heart rate are assessed. Adults severely affected may require intramuscular administration of atropine (0.4 mg). Contraindications include glaucoma and heart disease. However, we have never witnessed a vasovagal response to epidural injection that has not responded satisfactorily to conservative management.

C. The patient receives home care instructions, including a detailed description of potential complications related to infection. The patient signs the release form and a copy is given to the patient, which includes the phone contact numbers of the radiology department.

D. The patient is reassured that the effects of the injection will not be felt immediately and will gradually develop, with some relief beginning in approximately two to three days. The duration of the pain relief is difficult to assess before the injection and is highly individualized. We instruct the patient that benefits and results of the injection should be discussed with the referring physician, as sometimes a series of injections is required, whereas other times a single injection can provide therapeutic relief. A common patient statement is, "I was doing great after the injection I had on x date. Then I did x and my pain returned, so I came back hoping to get relief."

E. In the event of a wet tap with subsequent post-procedural headache, the patient may be required to receive a blood patch. This can be safely performed by the radiologist utilizing the lumbar approach. Approximately 20 ml of the patient's blood is obtained and 10–13 ml of the blood is injected into the epidural space at the site of the prior puncture. Strict adherence to sterile technique (mask, gown, and the like) is essential for the blood patch procedure.

IX. Procedure Reporting

A. The final epidural steroid injection report should include:
1. Patient name
2. Procedure (e.g., epidural steroid injection)
3. Date
4. Clinical history, including indication for the study (e.g., low back pain, neck pain, L4–5 radiculopathy, and the like)
5. Procedure technique
   a. Puncture site
   b. Name and amount of contrast agent
6. Findings
   a. Mention any incidentally noted abnormalities on the epidurogram
   b. Describe any complications (e.g., intrathecal injection, vasovagal response, allergic reaction)
7. Impression
   a. Describe if procedure was technically successful
   b. Mention if home care instructions were provided to the patient

X. Epidural Steroid Injection Coding

A. Procedural coding for epidural injection of steroids

	CPT Code
1. Cervical injection	62281
2. Lumbar injection	62282
B. Fluoroscopy charge (both approaches)	76000

SUGGESTED READING

1. Berman AT, Garbarino JL, Jr., Fisher SM, Bosacco SJ: The effects of epidural injection of local anesthetics and corticosteroids on patients with lumbosciatic pain. Clin Orthop 188:144–151, 1984.
2. Bush K, Cowan N, Katz DE, Gishen P: The natural history of sciatica associated with disc pathology: a prospective study with clinical and independent radiological follow-up. Spine 17:1205–1212, 1992.
3. Dilke TF, Burry HC, Grahame R: Extradural corticosteroid injection in management of lumbar nerve root compression. Br Med J 2:635–637, 1973.
4. El-Khoury GY, Ehara S, Weinstein JN, et al: Epidural steroid injection: a procedure ideally performed with fluoroscopic control. Radiology 168:554–557, 1988.
5. Link S, El-Khoury GY, et al: Percutaneous epidural and nerve block and percutaneous lumbar sympatholysis. Interventional Procedures in Musculoskeletal Radiology 1. Radiol Clin N Am 36:509–521, 1998.
6. Renfrew DL, Moore TE, Kathol MH, et al: Correct placement of epidural steroid injection: fluoroscopic guidance and contrast administration. AJNR 12:1003–1007, 1991.
7. Spaccarelli KC: Lumbar and caudal epidural corticosteroid injections. Mayo Clin Proceed 71:169–178, 1996.
8. Yates DW: Comparison of the types of epidural injection commonly used in the treatment of low back pain and sciatica. Rheumatol Rehab 17:181–186, 1978.

2

Spinal Nerve Blocks

Wade Wong, D.O.

Illustrations by

Daphne Theodorou, M.D.
and Stavroula Theodorou, M.D.

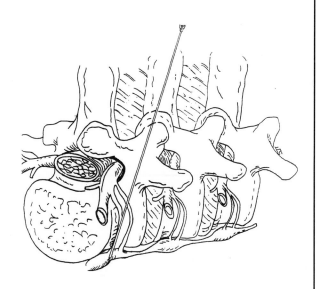

I. Types of Nerve Blocks

A. Direct nerve root blocks
  1. Lumbar postganglionic nerve blocks
  2. Lumbar periganglionic nerve blocks
  3. Thoracic nerve blocks
  4. Cervical nerve blocks
B. Indirect: epidural nerve blocks
  1. Midline or translaminar (paramedian)
  2. Transforaminal (essentially a periganglionic nerve block)
C. Facet joint blocks
  1. Intraarticular
  2. Medium branch blocks
D. Common sympathetic nerve blocks
  1. Stellate ganglion blockade
  2. Celiac plexus blockade
  3. Lumbar sympathetic blockade
  4. Impar ganglion blockade

II. Direct Nerve Blocks

A. Rationale
  1. Diagnostic: For diagnosis of radicular pain, especially when imaging is confusing.
  2. Therapeutic: applied to specific nerve following successful diagnostic nerve block. Local anesthetic and steroid are commonly used for therapy; other techniques such as neurolysis or radiofrequency ablation (see Chapter 3) may be considered for refractory cases.
B. Contraindications
  1. Allergy (relative, as patient could be premedicated)
  2. Superficial infection along the needle path
  3. Uncorrectable coagulopathy
  4. Contralateral pneumothorax (thoracic nerve block)
C. Informed consent: the patient should be informed of the possible risks, including allergy, bleeding, nerve injury, paralysis, adverse reaction to any of the medications, seizure, headache, cardiac arrest, infection, respiratory arrest.
D. Equipment and supplies
  1. Multidirectional fluoroscopy or CT

2. Sterile setup

3. Needles: 3½ in to 6 in needles, 22 to 25 gauge

4. Omnipaque 180 or 240

5. Lidocaine: 1–2%

6. Marcaine: 0.25% to 0.5%

7. Celestone Soluspan: 6 mg/ml

E. Pertinent anatomy

1. The nerve root exits the neural foramen in the thoracic and lumbar region just inferior to the adjacent pedicle.

2. The ganglion is situated along the lateral aspect of the neural foramen.

3. The postganglionic portion of the lumbar exiting nerve root passes slightly anteriorly and inferior laterally to cross just under the midsection of the next lower level transverse process (Fig. 2–1).

4. In the thoracic region the nerve root exits the neural foramen and passes along the inferior margin of the adjacent rib (Fig. 2–2).

5. In the cervical region, the nerve root passes out from the neural foramen and posterior to the vertebral artery. It then procedes inferiorly and slightly laterally.

6. In the sacral region, the sensory nerve roots pass dorsally through the posterior neural foramen, and the motor roots pass anteriorly through the corresponding anterior neural foramen.

F. Sedation

1. Local anesthetic (1% lidocaine) is administered into the skin and soft tissues along the path of the needle to the nerve root.

2. The patient's blood pressure, pulse, and oxygen saturation are monitored. Conscious sedation is usually not necessary.

G. Procedure

1. Lumbar postganglionic nerve blocks

a. Usually for diagnostic purposes.

b. Injection of the postganglionic portion of the nerve sheath can be performed with local anesthetic and with little risk of reflux into the subarachnoid space.

c. The nerve root leaves the neural foramen and passes anteriorly and inferior laterally, crossing the mid portion of the next lower level transverse process.

d. For a postganglionic nerve block, the patient should be placed in the prone position. With the fluoroscope in the AP plane, the

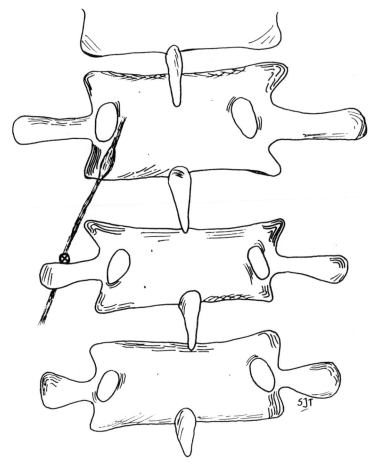

Figure 2–1. Postganglionic nerve block. The "X" within the small circle symbolizes vertical needle passage posterior to anterior to target.

superior aspect mid portion of the transverse process is targeted immediately inferior to the foramen of the desired nerve root.

e. After the patient is prepared, the local anesthetic is applied and a 22 to 25 gauge needle is passed just over the superior margin of the midsection of the transverse process just inferior to the concerned nerve root.

f. When a paresthesia is experienced by the patient, the needle is withdrawn barely 1 millimeter and iodinated contrast medium is injected to visualize contrast around the filling defect of the postganglionic portion of the nerve root (see Fig. 2–1).

g. For diagnostic blocks, 2–3 ml of 1% lidocaine is given.

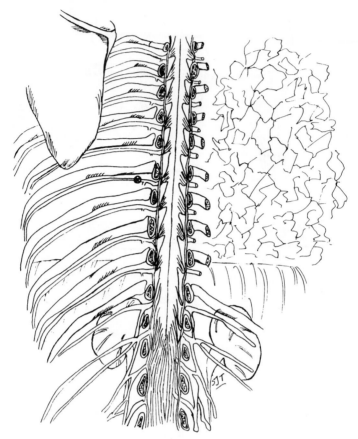

Figure 2-2. Thoracic nerve block. The "X" within the small circle symbolizes the target zone for the tip of the needle just inferior to the rib.

h. Therapeutic blockades can also be performed by injecting 2 ml of 1% lidocaine or Marcaine 0.25% and 1 ml of Celestone 6 mg/ml.

2. Lumbar periganglionic nerve blocks (transforaminal epidural steroid injection)

a. This procedure can be performed with either fluoroscopic or CT guidance. A C-arm fluoroscope is preferred.

b. From a posterior lateral and somewhat inferior to superior approach, a starting point is chosen to access the concerned neural foramen (Fig. 2–3*A*). The patient is prepared and draped.

c. Local anesthetic is administered below the skin surface and along the expected track of the path of the needle. A 22 or 25 gauge needle is directed to the neural foramen to contact the rostral pedicle at the 6:00 position.

d. On the AP view, the needle should not be passed any more medially than the medial border of the pedicle (Fig. 2–3*B*), otherwise the subarachnoid space may be encountered.

e. Iodinated contrast (2–3 ml of Omnipaque 180) is injected to define the nerve root as it exits the neural foramen.

f. Frequently there will be extension of contrast along the adjacent epidural space. Therefore, this technique can also be considered a transforaminal epidural steroid injection.

g. This technique is commonly utilized following a postganglionic diagnostic nerve block: 1 ml of lidocaine 1% or Marcaine 0.25% can be injected along with 1–2 ml of Celestone, 6 mg/ml, for therapy.

3. Thoracic nerve blocks

a. These procedures are usually performed along the immediate postganglionic segment as the nerve courses just inferior to the adjacent rib. C-arm fluoroscopy is necessary.

b. A starting point is chosen just inferior to the proximal rib immediately lateral to the neural foramen (see Fig. 2–2). The patient is placed in the prone position.

c. AP fluoroscopy is utilized to direct a needle along the proximal inferior portion of the rib to contact the intended nerve root.

d. Once the patient is prepped and draped, local anesthetic is injected along the path of the needle. When the needle is started in the AP plane, the fluoroscope is turned to the lateral plane to verify the depth and to avoid causing a pneumothorax.

e. A paresthesia is usually provoked when the needle contacts the nerve root.

f. Injection of 2–3 ml of iodinated contrast will outline the adjacent intercostal nerve proximally.

g. For diagnostic nerve blocks, 1–2 ml of lidocaine 1% (or Marcaine 0.25%) can be injected.

h. For therapeutic blockade, 1–2 ml of Celestone, 6 mg/ml, can be added.

i. It is extremely important to visualize the tip of the needle from the lateral view as it passes anteriorly in order to avoid causing a pneumothorax.

j. Also, arrangements for placement of a chest tube or a chest tube kit should be available when performing this procedure.

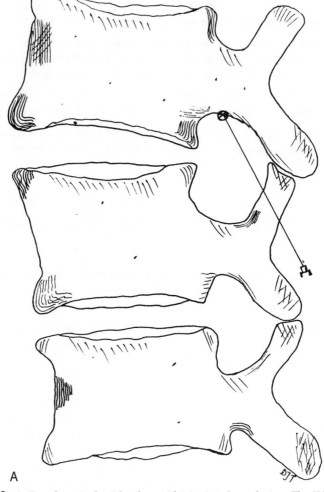

A

Figure 2–3. *A*, Transforaminal epidural steroid injection. Lateral view. The "X" within the small circle symbolizes the target zone for the tip of the needle.

4. Cervical nerve blocks
   a. Fluoroscopy or CT can be utilized in performing a cervical nerve block.
   b. The entry zone on the skin is lateral or slightly anterolateral to the neural foramen.
   c. Visualization of the neural foramen from this approach should be established by either CT or C-arm fluoroscopy. The patient is placed in the supine position and prepped and draped as usual.
   d. Local anesthetic is injected along the projected path of the subse-

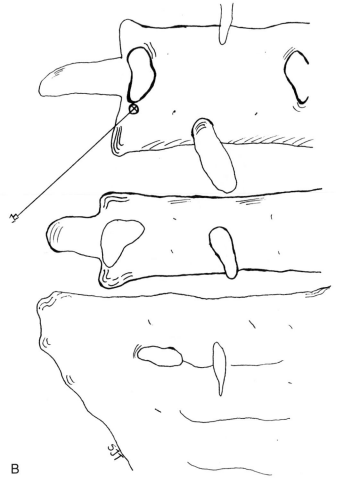

B

Figure 2–3 *Continued. B,* Transforaminal epidural steroid injection. Anteroposterior view. The "X" within the small circle symbolizes the target zone for the tip of the needle.

quent nerve block needle. A 22 to 25 gauge needle is directed to the posterior margin of the neural foramen with the needle aimed at the superior face (Fig. 2–4).

e. Once the needle reaches the posterior margin of the neural foramen, iodinated contrast material is injected (1–2 ml of Omnipaque 180) to outline the exiting nerve root ganglion complex.

f. It is important to stay along the posterior margin of the neural foramen to avoid injury to the adjacent vertebral artery, which is situated anterior to the neural foramen.

g. When injecting contrast, one should not normally observe filling

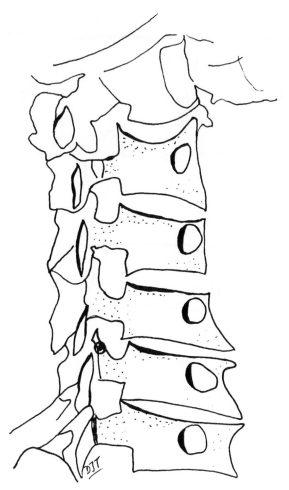

Figure 2–4. Lateral view seen at fluoroscopy in cervical nerve root block. The "X" within the small circle marks the bony landmark target for injection of the dorsal root at or just lateral to the ganglion, in this case at C5.

of the subarachnoid space, and there should never be vascular runoff.

    h. Once the needle is satisfactorily situated, injection of 1 ml lidocaine 1% can be done for diagnostic purposes and/or 1–2 ml of Celestone 6 mg/ml can be injected for therapeutic purposes.

H. Post-procedural care

    1. The patient is observed for 30 minutes before discharge.

    2. If a thoracic nerve block has been performed, special attention should paid to any unusual shortness of breath; this should prompt an expiratory chest x-ray to rule out pneumothorax.

3. The patient should be instructed to avoid driving and strenuous physical activity for 24 hours. The patient should be given a phone contact to use if there is any unusual pain, headache, fever, or shortness of breath.

I. Procedural reporting

1. Mention should always be made of the specifics of informed consent, prepping and draping, local anesthetic, guidance of the needle by CT or fluoroscopy, and the size and type of the needle. Was there a paresthesia or a pain response identical to the patient's original pain when the needle tip contacted the nerve?

2. Permanent record confirmation of needle placement by injection of iodinated contrast must be made with hard copy or digital imaging.

3. The dosage and type of pharmaceutical injected should be recorded. Did a complication occur?

4. Mention should be made of any reduction in the level of pain following the procedure.

5. Finally, if you believe that the patient may benefit from a repeat block, this should be communicated to the referring physician.

III. Indirect Spinal Nerve Blocks: Epidural Injection

See the section on epidural injections for techniques concerning midline, translaminar, transforaminal, and caudal approaches.

IV. Facet Joint Block

See the section on facet injections and median branch nerve blocks.

V. Common Sympathetic Nerve Blocks

A. Stellate ganglion blockade

1. Indications

a. Reflex sympathetic dystrophy of the upper extremity

b. Raynaud's syndrome of the upper extremity or painful upper extremity as a result of arterial insufficiency, including chronic arterial emboli

c. Herpes zoster of the face, neck, and upper thorax

d. Posttraumatic syndrome: swelling, excessive sweating

e. Hyperhydrosis of the upper extremity and neck

2. Contraindications

a. Uncorrectable coagulopathy

b. Contralateral pneumothorax

c. Recent myocardial infarction (accelerator nerves to the heart pass through the stellate ganglion; therefore, a sympathetic blockade may result in heart block or bradycardia with diminished cardiac output)

d. Glaucoma

3. Informed consent: it should be explained that complications can include intravascular injection, bleeding, air embolism, diaphragmatic paralysis due to close proximity to the phrenic nerve, hoarseness (due to close proximity to the recurrent laryngeal nerve), pneumothorax, hypotension, bradycardia, intraspinal injection (paralysis, seizures).

4. Pertinent anatomy

a. The stellate ganglion is the fusion of the most inferior cervical ganglion and the most superior thoracic ganglion.

b. It is situated deep and in close proximity to the vertebral artery, and medial and posterior to the carotid artery and the jugular vein.

c. This large, flat ganglion is a key relay station (synapse or pass through) of sympathetic nerves of the head and neck as well as of the upper extremity.

d. The target zone for needle placement is the lateral border of the C7 vertebra at its juncture with the transverse process.

5. Equipment and supplies:

a. Biplane fluoroscopy (CT also acceptable).

b. Local anesthesia with lidocaine along the needle path.

c. 25 gauge spinal needle to access the stellate ganglion.

d. Iodinated contrast (Omnipaque 180).

e. Anesthetic can be either lidocaine 1% or 2% for diagnosis, for longer effect (2–6 days) Marcaine 0.25%, or, for neurolysis, absolute alcohol or phenol 6%.

6. Sedation: awake or mild oral hypnotics as necessary

7. Procedure

a. The patient is placed in the supine position.

b. Fluoroscopic localization takes place along the AP plane for the target zone along the lateral border of the C7 vertebral body at the junction with the proximal aspect of the ipsilateral transverse process (Fig. 2–5).

c. Some nonradiologists target Chassaignac's tubercle (lateral border of C6) by palpation for needle placement.

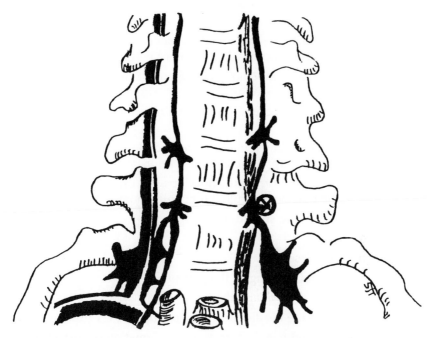

Figure 2–5. Anatomic location of sympathetic chains and stellate ganglia (dark, thick structures) in the neck, with relationship to bony anatomic landmarks illustrated as would be seen under fluoroscopy.

d. The patient is prepped and draped. Local anesthetic is injected just below the skin surface and along the intended path of the needle.

e. A 25 gauge needle is directed vertically down along an AP plane to reach the lateral border of the C7 vertebral body where the transverse process arises (see Fig. 2–5). The needle should be aspirated to rule out intravascular location when it has been positioned.

f. Iodinated contrast (2–3 ml of Omnipaque 180) should be injected to rule out intravascular or intraspinal communication and to verify needle tip location.

g. For pain management, Marcaine 0.25% (10 ml) may be injected as often as once a week.

h. For neurolysis, 10 ml of absolute alcohol is the agent of choice currently and can be slowly injected. This should be performed with either very heavy conscious sedation or general anesthesia, because injection of alcohol can be very painful.

i. The needle is removed and direct pressure is applied for a few (5–10) minutes.

8. Post-procedure care
   a. After successful stellate ganglion blockade, Horner's syndrome (ptosis, myosis, and nasal congestion) is common.
   b. There may also be venous engorgement or paresthesias in the ipsilateral upper extremity.
   c. Hoarseness may occur if the nearby recurrent laryngeal nerve is anesthetized.
   d. The patient should remain in the radiology department under observation for approximately one hour.
   e. If any shortness of breath develops, an expiratory chest x-ray should be obtained to rule out pneumothorax.

9. Procedure reporting should include:
   a. Indications
   b. Informed consent
   c. Prepping and draping of the patient
   d. Application of local anesthetic
   e. Direction of the needle under fluoroscopic or CT guidance
   f. Injection of iodinated contrast for confirmation of correct needle placement (and the lack of intravascular or intraspinal communication)
   g. Injection of pharmaceuticals
   h. Any complications
   i. Results

B. Celiac plexus blockade
   1. Indications
      a. Intractable pain in the upper abdomen from pancreatic cancer or chronic pancreatitis
      b. Upper abdominal chronic pain from deep visceral arterial insufficiency
      c. Chronic pain from the distal esophagus, stomach, upper small bowel, transverse colon, adrenals, spleen, or liver
   2. Contraindications
      a. Bowel obstruction—there may be increased motility with uncontested parasympathetic innervation as a result of sympathetic denervation
      b. Uncorrected coagulopathy
      c. Local superficial subcutaneous infection along the course of the needle
      d. Allergy to any of the medications

3. Informed consent: as for other procedures
4. Pertinent anatomy: celiac ganglia are situated on either side of the celiac arterial trunk and are located anterior to the crura of the diaphragm.
5. Equipment and supplies
   a. CT scan (alternative: ultrasound guidance)
   b. Needles for local anesthesia (lidocaine 1%) and 3½ in to 6 in 22 or 25 gauge needles to reach the celiac ganglia for treatment
   c. Medications include lidocaine, iodinated contrast agent (Omnipaque 180 or 240), and Marcaine 0.25%.
   d. For neurolysis, absolute alcohol should be used.
6. Conscious sedation
   a. For temporary blockade with Marcaine, conscious sedation is optional.
   b. Heavy conscious sedation or general anesthesia is recommended for neurolysis with absolute alcohol administration.
7. Procedure
   a. The patient is placed in the prone position for a posterior to anterior approach.
   b. Initial CT sections should be obtained at approximately the T12 level to locate the celiac artery.
   c. The patient is prepped and draped in the usual sterile manner.
   d. Local anesthetic is applied with skin entry sites starting slightly lateral to the spinous process of the vertebra (approximately 5–7 cm) because the needle's course is along the posteriolateral aspect of the adjacent vertebra with lateral to medial angulation.
   e. Slightly caudal gantry angulation will aid in avoiding the inferior margins of the lungs and medial aspect of the diaphragms posteriorly.
   f. Following local anesthetic administration, 22 gauge needles are directed along the sides of the adjacent vertebral body and directed anteriorly so that they are positioned just anterior to the aorta passing through the crura.
   g. The needle tip will be adjacent to the celiac artery (Fig. 2–6).
   h. It may be necessary to place needles bilaterally so that needle tips bracket both sides of the celiac artery anterior to the crura of the diaphragm.
   i. It may occasionally be necessary to pass a needle through the aorta.
   j. Contrast material is then injected to verify the lack of intravascu-

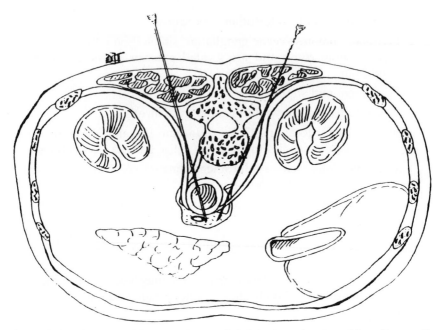

Figure 2-6. Illustration of CT slice of upper abdomen shows location of the celiac ganglion and two alternative approaches with needles under CT guidance. Note that approaching from the left side of the back necessitates transit through the aorta. The celiac ganglion is not a well-defined anatomic structure, even on the highest resolution CT images.

lar communication and to observe the expected distribution of the medications on either side of the celiac artery and the lack of retrocrural communication.

  k. Injection of 10 ml of Marcaine 0.25% is performed in a slow, progressive manner for temporary pain relief.

  l. For neurolysis, approximately 10 ml of absolute alcohol can be injected under general anesthesia or heavy conscious sedation. Injection of absolute alcohol can be extremely painful.

8. Alternative procedure

  a. Anterior to posterior needle passage through the left lobe of the liver can be performed with CT or ultrasound guidance.

  b. The patient is placed in the supine position.

  c. The celiac artery is located by appropriate imaging (CT or ultrasound).

  d. The patient is prepped and draped and local anesthetic is administered.

  e. A 22 or 25 gauge needle is directed through the left lobe of the liver so that the tip is situated beside the celiac artery.

f. Iodinated contrast is injected to confirm the needle tip location.

g. Medications as noted previously are injected into or around the celiac ganglia.

9. Post-procedural care

   a. The patient is kept in the recovery room for 4 hours with vital sign monitoring.

   b. The patient should be monitored for sudden onset of hypotension due to pooling of blood in the gastrointestinal circulation after release of parasympathetic tone associated with neural blockade.

   c. This can be treated with generous IV fluids usually for up to 24 hours.

   d. Hypotension may last for 2–3 days and may require hospitalization.

   e. The patient should be monitored for bleeding, particularly if a transaortic or transhepatic route is taken.

10. Reporting: as in other interventional procedures previously mentioned.

C. Lumbar sympathetic blockade

1. Indications

   a. Reflex sympathetic dystrophy of the lower extremities

   b. Phantom limb pain, frostbite

   c. Trench foot, gangrene of the feet

   d. Pain from arterial insufficiency due to Raynaud's syndrome or chronic arterial emboli

   e. Hyperhydrosis of the lower extremities

   f. Chronic renal colic

2. Contraindications

   a. Uncorrected coagulopathy

   b. Subcutaneous infection along the course of the needle

   c. Allergy

3. Informed consent: risks include intravascular injection, genital femoral neuralgia, psoas necrosis, ureteral injury, hypotension, impotence, bleeding.

4. Pertinent anatomy

   a. The lumbar sympathetic ganglia are located anterior and lateral to the vertebral body from L2 to L5.

   b. The target zone for this injection is located along the anterior lateral aspects of the L2 vertebra.

5. Equipment and supplies
   a. Fluoroscopy, preferably multidirectional C-arm. Alternative is CT guidance.
   b. Local anesthesia with lidocaine and the use of appropriate needles for local anesthetic.
   c. 25 or 22 gauge long needles usually 3½ in to 6 in
   d. Marcaine 0.25% (or absolute alcohol for neurolysis)

6. Sedation: local anesthetic is usually adequate for most cases unless neurolysis with absolute alcohol is to be peformed, in which case heavy conscious sedation or general anesthesia would be indicated for pain management.

7. Procedure
   a. The patient is placed in the prone position.
   b. Fluoroscopic or CT targeting is done in such a way that the needle tip is situated along the anterolateral aspect of the L2 vertebra.
   c. The patient is prepped and draped and local anesthetic is administered in the usual manner.
   d. A 22 or 25 gauge spinal needle is directed from posterior to anterior and from lateral to medial so that the tip of the needle is finally situated along the anterolateral aspect of the L2 vertebra (Fig. 2–7). Iodinated contrast is injected to confirm needle tip location and the absence of intravascular communication (particularly into the aorta or inferior vena cava).
   e. For therapy, injection of 10 ml of 0.25% Marcaine is performed for temporary relief, usually lasting up to one week.
   f. Injections for reflex sympathetic dystrophy may be repeated on a weekly basis for up to 6–8 weeks.
   g. For neurolysis, absolute alcohol is injected in the same technical manner as already noted (10 ml).

8. Post-procedural care: patient is observed for about 2 hours for any potential complications. The patient should arrange to be driven home.

9. Reporting: as in other interventional procedures mentioned previously.

D. Impar ganglion blockade
   1. Indications: intractable low pelvic and perineal pain usually resulting from rectal cancer, uterine cancer, prostate cancer, endometriosis, or adhesions of the lower bowel
   2. Contraindications: similar to the lumbar sympathetic blockades

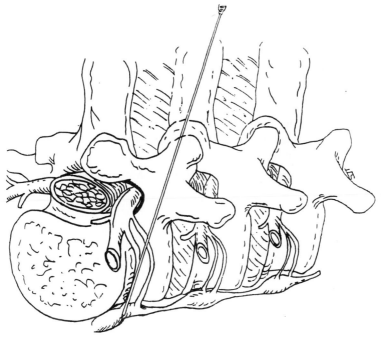

Figure 2-7. Needle optimally positioned in the left sympathetic ganglion anterolateral to the L2 vertebral body, as viewed from above.

3. Informed consent: risks include infection, bleeding, nerve injury

4. Pertinent anatomy: the impar ganglion runs along the anterior surface of the sacrum just posterior to the rectum and close to the midline; it is the ganglion in which the sympathetic trunks of the two sides unite

5. Equipment and supplies

   a. Fluoroscopy (multidirectional C-arm)

   b. Appropriate needles for local anesthetic along with 1% lidocaine and contrast agent (Omnipaque 180)

   c. Marcaine or absolute alcohol for neurolytic ablation

6. Sedation: as noted previously

7. Procedure

   a. The patient is in the prone position.

   b. Target the anterior surface of the sacrum with the fluoroscope, observing in the lateral view.

   c. The patient is prepared and draped as usual, with a local anesthetic applied to the starting point just under the coccyx.

    d. A 22 gauge spinal needle that has been pre-bent at a 30-degree angle is used; usually two bends are adequate.

    e. The needle is directed immediately posterior so that the tip reaches the anterior surface of the sacrum (Fig. 2–8).

    f. The C-arm fluoroscope is turned to view in the AP plane and the needle should appear to be in the midline.

    g. An iodinated contrast agent is injected, and the contrast should be seen to layer along the anterior surface of the sacrum and not in the rectum.

    h. For temporary pain relief, 10 ml of Marcaine 0.25% is injected.

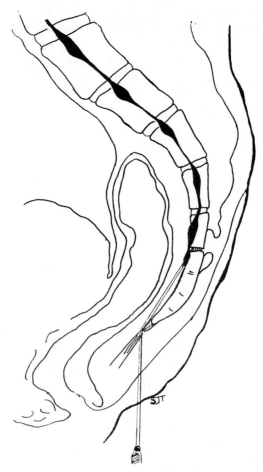

Figure 2–8. The lateral view of the sacrum as seen with fluoroscopy when approaching the impar ganglion. The needle has a 30 degree dorsal bend so that the tip is positioned adjacent to the ventral periosteum of the sacrum.

   i. Neurolysis, which should be performed under heavy conscious sedation or general anesthesia, requires 10 ml of absolute alcohol, which should be injected slowly.

8. Post-procedural care: similar to lumbar sympathetic blockades

9. Reporting: as in other interventional procedures mentioned already.

VI. Procedural Coding

	CPT Code
A. Cervical nerve blocks	
1. Lumbar nerve block	64440
2. Lumbar neurolytic nerve block	64640
3. Intercostal nerve block single level	64420
4. Multiple levels	64421
5. Neurolytic blockade	64620
B. Stellate ganglion blockade	64510
C. Neurolytic blockade	64680
D. Celiac plexus blockade	64530
Neurolytic blockade	64680
E. Lumbar sympathetic blockade	64520
Neurolytic blockade	64640
F. Impar ganglion blockade	64999
Neurolytic blockade	64640

SUGGESTED READING

1. Erickson SJ, Hogan QH: CT guided injection of the stellate ganglion: description of technique and efficacy of sympathetic blockade. Radiology 188:707–709, 1993.
2. Gangi A, Dietemann JL, Mortazavi R, et al: CT-guided interventional procedures for pain management in the lumbosacral spine. Radiographics 18:621–633, 1998.
3. Gangi A, Dietemann JL, Schultz A, et al: Interventional radiologic procedures with CT guidance, Cancer Pain Management. Radiographics 16:1289–1304, 1996.
4. Gimenez A, Martinez-Noguera A, Donoso L, et al: Percutaneous neurolysis of the celiac plexus via anterior approach with sonographic guidance. AJR 161:1061–1063, 1993.
5. Vall'ee JN, Feydy A, Carlier RY, et al: Chronic cervical radiculopathy: lateral-approach periradicular cortico-steroid injection. Radiology 218:886–892, 2001.
6. Waldman SD: Atlas of Interventional Pain Management. Philadelphia, WB Saunders, 1998.
7. Waldman SD, Winnie AP: Interventional Pain Management. Philadelphia, WB Saunders, 1996, pp 269–271.
8. Wong W: Management of back pain using image guidance. J Women's Imaging 2:88–97, 2000.
9. Zennaro H, Dousset V, Viand B, et al: Periganglionic foraminal steroid injections performed under CT control. AJNR 19:349–352, 1998.
10. Murtagh R: The art and science of nerve root and facit block. Neuroimag Clin North Am 10:465–477, 2000.

3

Pulsed Radiofrequency Techniques in Clinical Practice

Farshad M. Ahadian, M.D.

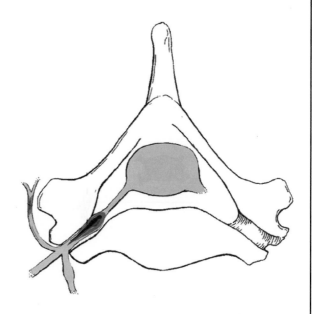

I. Rationale and Clinical Indications

A. Radiofrequency ablation (RFA) may be used for selective neuroablative procedures for treatment of various chronic pain disorders. More recently, the advent of pulsed radiofrequency ablation (PRFA) has made this treatment safer, which has significantly increased its utility. *PRFA is recommended for all lesions discussed in Chapter 2.*

B. Conventional RFA at higher temperatures (80–90°C) is best avoided for many nerve root and peripheral nerve lesions due to risk of neuroma formation and worsening neuropathic pain.

C. PRFA used in a temperature range of 40–45°C appears to be just as effective as conventional RFA without the associated risks.

D. All neurolytic techniques, including RFA and PRFA, must be preceded by diagnostic/prognostic local anesthetic and possibly corticosteroid nerve blocks to identify the appropriate spinal segment involved and to assess the potential benefit from long-term neurolysis.

Advantages of PRFA over other neuroablative techniques:

a. Produces quantifiable lesions

b. Avoids sticking and charring

c. Minimal soft tissue trauma

d. No gas formation

e. Allows impedance monitoring

f. Neurostimulation capability prior to lesion

g. Small, easy to use needle

h. Electrode amenable to stereotactic and fluoroscopy-guided procedures

i. Electrodes may be made very sturdy and in various shapes and configurations

II. Contraindications and Informed Consent

A. Lack of informed consent

B. Infection at the site of the procedure

C. Systemic infection

D. Coagulopathy

E. Platelet dysfunction

F. Severe cardiopulmonary disease (relative contraindication for procedures in the cervical and thoracic regions)

G. The risks for infection, bleeding, nerve trauma, paralysis, allergic reactions, headache, adverse cardiac and pulmonary events, as well as worsening of pain, should be discussed with the patient before all of these procedures.

H. In addition, special complications listed in each section should be discussed in detail.

III. Equipment and Supplies

A. C-arm fluoroscopy

B. Sterile setup

C. Lidocaine 0.5–1.0% for local anesthesia

D. Iohexol (Omnipaque) 180 or 240

E. RF generator with pulse-mode capability

F. RF probe (5, 10, or 15 cm lengths)

G. RF insulated needles (22 or 23 gauge; 5, 10, or 15 cm lengths; 4 or 10 mm active tips)

IV. Pertinent Anatomy

See in sections on individual procedures.

V. Anesthesia and Sedation

A. *Sedation*

1. Because of limitations in local anesthesia and duration of procedures, some patients may require conscious sedation.

2. Heavy sedation must be avoided, as patient cooperation is necessary for the success of the procedure.

B. *Local anesthesia*

1. Infiltration of local anesthetics should be limited to the skin and very superficial soft tissue.

2. 0.5–1.0% lidocaine or similar agent is adequate for anesthetizing the superficial structures.

3. Deeper infiltration will interfere with neurostimulation and may cause difficulty with needle positioning and poor outcome.

VI. Radiofrequency Procedures

A. Neurostimulation

1. Sensory and motor stimulation prior to a PRFA lesion is recommended for both safety and success of the procedure; 50 Hertz (Hz) frequency is used first for sensory stimulation.

2. The intensity of stimulation is increased slowly until the patient acknowledges the onset of cramping, aching, or tingling in an area corresponding to the neural structure targeted.

3. The voltage at which the patient first perceives the stimulation is the *sensory threshold*. The lower the sensory threshold, the closer the tip of the needle is to the targeted nerve.

4. If the perceived area of stimulation does not match the targeted nerve distribution clinically, further radiographic examination is warranted and the needle tip should be adjusted appropriately. The frequency is then changed to 2 Hz for motor stimulation.

5. The intensity is increased to two to three times the voltage for sensory threshold. There should be no motor activity in the distribution of nearby somatic nerves.

6. At this point the RF machine is switched to "Pulsed Mode" and the PRFA lesion is induced.

B. The PRFA Lesion

1. The optimal duration of the PRFA lesion is not known. Total lesion times as short as 1 minute and as long as 6 minutes have been used successfully.

2. The distance from the RF probe to the nerve structure and the diameter of the nerve as well as the vascularity of the surrounding structures are some of the variables that may affect the success of the lesion.

3. The current recommendation is 2–4 minutes.

4. The other lesion parameters include frequency of the current used to induce the lesion itself (2 Hz) and the duration of each pulse (20 msec).

5. The voltage output is increased until the temperature reaches 40–45°C.

C. Special neurotomy procedures

1. Cervical medial branch PRFA

   a. Indications

      (1) Cervical facet arthropathy

      (2) Cervicogenic headaches

   b. Pertinent Anatomy (Figs. 3–1 and 3–2)

      (1) The C3-4 to C7-T1 facet joints are innervated by the medial branches of the cervical dorsal rami at the same level as the joint and from the segment immediately above.

      (2) The medial branches originate in the cervical intertransverse

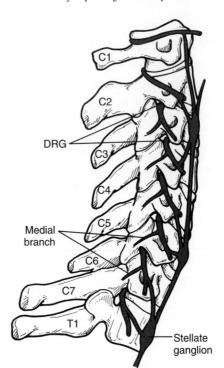

Figure 3-1. Lateral view of the cervical spine. Note the location of the dorsal root ganglion (DRG) within each neural foramen, as well as the medial branches of the dorsal primary rami of C3-C7. The sympathetic chain and the three cervical ganglia are also depicted along the anterolateral aspect of the vertebral bodies.

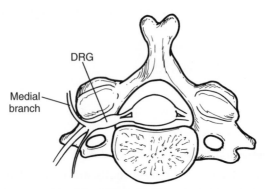

Figure 3-2. Cross sectional view of cervical vertebra. Note the location of the DRG within the neural foramen as well as the medial branch of the dorsal primary ramus.

spaces and then wrap around the concave areas, or waists, of their respective articular pillars.

(3) The medial branch of the C8 dorsal ramus crosses the root of the T1 transverse process. Instead of wrapping around an articular pillar, it hooks medially onto the lamina of T1, sending articular branches to the C7-T1 facet joint.

(4) The C2-3 facet joint differs in that it is innervated by the C2 posterior rami as well as by the large third occipital nerve, which is one of the two medial branches from the C3 dorsal ramus.

(5) The atlanto-occipital and lateral atlantoaxial joints are not innervated by the cervical posterior rami; instead, they receive branches from the C1 and C2 ventral rami.

c. Procedure

(1) Both posterior and lateral approaches to the cervical medial branches have been described.

(2) The posterior approach with the patient in the prone position is favored due to its lower risk of penetration of the vertebral artery, the epidural space, or the dural sac. The posterior approach will be described here.

   a. For the majority of the patients, a 54 mm RF needle provides adequate length to reach the targets. For morbidly obese patients, a longer needle may be used. A 4 mm active tip is recommended for the cervical region.

   b. For C3-8 medial branch PRFA, the cervical spine should first be examined under anteroposterior (AP) view of fluoroscopy.

   c. A 22 or 23 gauge insulated RF needle is inserted in line or slightly lateral (3–5 mm) to the lateral concavity, or the waist, of the articular pillar. The needle is advanced until the dorsal surface of the articular pillar is contacted.

   d. The tip is then redirected, or "walked off," laterally until the tip just slides off the edge.

   e. The tip should be advanced 3–5 mm so that the entire active tip of the needle is in contact with the periosteum. Care should be taken to avoid advancing the needle too far.

   f. Needle position is then confirmed with lateral projection fluoroscopy.

(3) For the C2-C3 facet joint, the third occipital nerve is treated with PRFA in a manner similar to that for the medial branches

just discussed. The nerve is encountered at the lower half of the lateral margin of the C2-C3 facet.

2. Lumbar Medial Branch PRFA

   a. Indication: Lumbar facet arthropathy

   b. Pertinent Anatomy (Figs. 3–3 and 3–4)

      (1) In the lumbar region, the medial branch of the dorsal ramus lies in a groove formed at the base of the superior articular process of the facet joint.

      (2) The nerve passes in a dorsal and caudal direction, first innervating the joint capsule at the same level and then sending fibers to the next lower facet joint.

      (3) At the L5 level the transverse process is replaced by the ala of the sacrum.

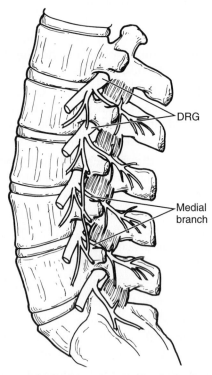

Figure 3–3. Lateral view of the lumbar spine. Notice the location of the DRG within the neural foramina from L1-L5. Also notice the course of the medial branches of the dorsal primary rami as they cross the junction of the transverse processes and the superior articular processes at each level. At the L5-S1 level the ala of the sacrum replaces the transverse processes.

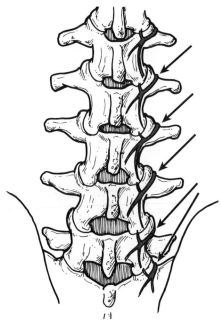

Figure 3–4. Posterior view of the lumbar spine. The medial branches are depicted in black. The arrows point to the target for PRFA lesion.

c. Procedure

(1) The patient is placed in the prone position with pillows beneath the abdomen to flatten the lumbar lordosis. The spine is examined under AP view of the fluoroscope.

(2) The cephalad/caudad angle of the C-arm is adjusted until the fluoroscope beam is parallel to the endplates of the vertebral body.

(3) The C-arm is then angulated obliquely 5–10 degrees ipsilateral to the medial branch to be treated. Using this view, the junction of the pedicle, the superior articulating process, and the transverse process are easily visualized.

(4) Note that at the L5-S1 level, the ala of the sacrum replaces the transverse process.

(5) The needle is inserted into the skin at a point directly in line with this junction along the x-ray beam: that is, the needle is "gun barreled" toward the target.

(6) To decrease risk of trauma to the nerve root, the needle is first advanced until it contacts the superior articulating process.

(7) The tip is then "walked off" laterally until the active tip lies in the gutter formed by the superior articulating process and the transverse process.

    (8) The needle should be advanced slowly and if paresthesias are elicited, it should be slightly withdrawn.

3. Sacral Lateral Branch PRFA

  a. Indication: Sacroiliac arthropathy

  b. Pertinent Anatomy

    (1) The primary innervation of the sacroiliac joint is derived from the medial branch of the L5 dorsal ramus and the lateral branches of the S1 and S2 dorsal rami.

    (2) In some cases the L3 and L4 dorsal rami may also contribute to the sacroiliac joint innervation.

  c. Procedure

    (1) Analgesia for the sacroiliac joint may be obtained by PRFA of the medial branch of the L5 dorsal ramus and the lateral branches of S1 and S2 dorsal rami.

    (2) PRFA of the L5 medial branch is described under lumbar medial branch PRFA.

    (3) For the S1 and S2 medial branches, the sacrum should be visualized using an AP view of the fluoroscope. Cephalad/caudad angulation of the image intensifier is used until the sacral foramina are well visualized.

    (4) The needle is then passed under fluoroscopic guidance to contact the lateral angle of the external sacral foramen. The periosteum should be contacted first, immediately lateral to the foramen.

    (5) The needle is then "walked off" medially until the tip just falls into the neural foramen. There is no need to advance the needle into the foramen.

    (6) The medial branch is intercepted just as it exits the lateral angle of the foramen.

4. Dorsal Root Ganglion (DRG) PRFA

  a. Indications

    (1) Radiculitis

    (2) Peripheral nerve lesions

  b. Pertinent Anatomy (see Figs. 3–1 through 3–4)

    (1) Although the size and length of the DRG varies with vertebral level, the ganglion is generally located in the dorsal cephalad quadrant of the neural foramina.

    (2) In 90% of cases, the center of the ganglion lies directly caudad to the vertebral pedicle. In 8% of cases, the DRG is located

inferolateral to the pedicle, and in 2% of cases, it is medial to the pedicle within the lateral recess.

c. Procedure

  (1) Cervical DRG-PRFA

    a. The C3-C8 DRG may be accessed either in the supine position with a lateral needle approach or in the prone position with a dorsal oblique approach.

    b. In either case the needle tip is advanced to enter the dorsal cephalad quadrant of the neural foramina.

    c. Needle tip position should be checked under lateral fluoroscopy view to confirm correct placement within the foramen.

    d. The fluoroscope is then switched to the AP view and the needle advanced until the tip is in line with the mid-point of the pedicles. Note that the subarachnoid space and the vertebral artery are within easy reach.

    e. The needle should be advanced carefully and negative aspiration should be confirmed.

  (2) Lumbar DRG PRFA

    a. The patient is placed in the prone position. A 10–20 degree oblique view of the fluoroscope is used.

    b. A 10–15 cm needle with bent tip is recommended.

    c. The needle is directed just caudal to the pedicle and transverse process and advanced until the tip contacts the superior articulating process.

    d. The needle is then "walked off" ventrally until the tip enters the neural foramen.

    e. The lateral view of the fluoroscope is then used to confirm correct position of the needle tip in the dorsal-cephalad quadrant of the foramen.

    f. The fluoroscope is then changed to AP view, and the needle is advanced until the tip is in line with the mid-point of the pedicles.

    g. After satisfactory sensory and motor stimulation has been performed, a PRFA lesion is made.

  (3) Thoracic DRG PRFA

    a. The approach to the thoracic DRG is similar to the lumbar region but complicated by two structures: Laterally the lung is at risk of pneumothorax and dorsolaterally the ribs may impede access to the neural foramina.

     b. To minimize the risk of pneumothorax, the dorsal oblique angle of approach should be no more than 5–10 degrees from the sagittal plane. A 20 degree curve at the tip of the needle is instrumental in entering the neural foramen.

     c. The superior lateral edge of the thoracic lamina should first be contacted immediately caudal to the pedicle.

     d. The needle tip is then gently "walked off" laterally and advanced into the neural foramen.

     e. The C-arm is changed to lateral view and needle tip placement is confirmed within the dorsal-cephalad quadrant.

5. Stellate Ganglion PRFA

  a. Indications

    (1) Complex regional pain syndrome (CRPS)

    (2) Circulatory insufficiency

    (3) Hyperhidrosis

  b. Pertinent Anatomy (Fig. 3–5)

    (1) The cervicothoracic sympathetic ganglion lies in the space bounded dorsally by the prevertebral fascia and ventrally by the carotid sheath.

    (2) The lower cervical and first thoracic ganglia may be either separate or they may fuse to form the stellate ganglion, a diffuse structure overlying the anterolateral aspect of the C7 vertebral body and the neck of the first rib.

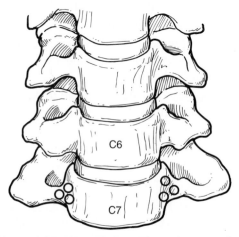

Figure 3–5. Anterior view of the cervical spine. The circles target the site for PRFA lesion of the cervical sympathetic chain using the anterior approach at C7.

c. Procedure

  (1) The patient is placed in the supine position. A 54 mm needle with a 4 mm active tip is used.

  (2) Three lesions are made in a triangular formation. Two lesions are made on the junction of the vertebral body with the transverse process: one lesion on the cephalad corner and another on the caudad corner of the vertebral body.

  (3) The third point is located more laterally on the transverse process of C7, approximately halfway in between the other two points. This pattern generates a triangular zone of interruption of the sympathetic fibers.

  (4) The needle is passed under fluoroscopic guidance to contact the periosteum at each of the points just described.

  (5) The needle is then pulled back 2 mm to ensure that the active tip is ventral to the longus colli muscle.

  (6) Proper sensory and motor stimulation prior to lesioning is important to avoid injury to the phrenic nerve, the recurrent laryngeal nerve, and the cervical plexus.

  (7) *Stimulation technique:* The following stimulation protocol should be performed prior to lesioning.

    a. First, sensory stimulation at 50 Hz and 2 volts should be negative.

    b. Next, motor stimulation at 2 Hz and 2.5 volts is performed while the patient pronounces the letter E. There should be no impairment in the patient's ability to articulate.

    c. If there is an impairment, the needle is anterior and medial to the target, in close proximity to the recurrent laryngeal nerve.

    d. Concurrently, a hand is placed on the subcostal region. Any movement of the diaphragm indicates the needle tip to be lateral to the target, adjacent to the phrenic nerve.

    e. Finally, sensory and motor stimulation of the upper extremity should be negative.

d. Specific Complications

  (1) Hematoma from vertebral artery, carotid artery, or jugular vein puncture

  (2) Neuralgia of brachial plexus or chest wall

  (3) Injury to the phrenic or recurrent laryngeal nerve

  (4) Pneumothorax

  (5) Horner's syndrome (rare)

(6) Osteitis (esophageal puncture)

6. Thoracic Sympathetic Chain PRFA

   a. Indications

      (1) Complex regional pain syndrome (CRPS)

      (2) Circulatory insufficiency

      (3) Hyperhidrosis

   b. Pertinent Anatomy

      (1) Complete sympathetic blockade of the upper extremity is difficult to achieve by treating the stellate ganglion alone. Blockade of the upper thoracic ganglia may be necessary.

      (2) The upper thoracic sympathetic chain is continuous with the cervical chain. It lies more dorsally, near the junction of the ventral two thirds and the dorsal one third of the vertebral body, adjacent to the periosteum.

      (3) The chain is in close proximity of the neck of the ribs, the somatic nerve roots, and the pleura.

   c. Procedure

      (1) Neurolysis of the upper thoracic sympathetic chain is generally performed at T2 and T3 levels. Both of these segments provide significant innervation to the upper extremity.

      (2) The patient is placed in the prone position.

      (3) AP view of the fluoroscope is initially selected. Cephalad angulation is then added until the fluoroscope beam is parallel to the superior and inferior endplates of T2 vertebral body. The T1-2 and T2-3 interspaces should be seen clearly using this view.

      (4) The C-arm is further angled obliquely so that a point just medial to the angle of each rib is in line (superimposed over) the edge of its respective vertebral body.

      (5) With a radiopaque pointer, the skin is marked in line with the other two points. This is the skin entry site.

      (6) The starting point should be slightly medial to the angle of the ribs to decrease the risk of pneumothorax

      (7) A 10 cm needle with a 10 mm active tip is used. Use of curved blunt-tip needles should be considered, as they may further decrease the risk of pneumothorax.

      (8) The needle is advanced parallel to the fluoroscopy beam. It should pass just under the inferior margin of the rib and contact the lateral edge of the vertebral body, first at T2 then at T3.

(9) As many as three lesions may be made at each vertebral level: the point described above, a point 3–5 mm cephalad, and another point 3–5 mm caudad.

(10) Because of the proximity of the somatic nerves, appropriate stimulation prior to lesioning is imperative.

(11) Patients may experience a deep aching sensation in the chest and back during stimulation and lesioning.

(12) Seven to 10 days of postoperative discomfort may be expected, and about 15% have a burning sensation in the upper chest wall for 1–2 weeks.

(13) A chest radiograph should be considered prior to discharge. However, because pneumothorax may not be radiographically apparent for 24 hours, the patient should be counseled to seek medical care if dyspnea or pleuritic pain occurs.

d. Specific Complications

(1) Pneumothorax

(2) Temporary chest and upper back discomfort

7. Lumbar Sympathetic Chain PRFA

a. Indications

(1) Complex regional pain syndrome (CRPS)

(2) Circulatory insufficiency

(3) Hyperhidrosis

b. Pertinent Anatomy (Fig. 3–6)

(1) In the lumbar region, the sympathetic chain and its ganglia extend along the ventrolateral aspect of the L1-L5 vertebral bodies. There is some anatomical variability, but the chain always lies ventral to the psoas sheath, which separates it from the somatic nerves.

(2) The aorta and vena cava lie just anterior to the body of the vertebra, and the ureters and somatic nerves are also in close proximity.

c. Procedure

(1) The procedure may be performed in the prone or lateral position. Most pain practitioners prefer to lesion the sympathetic chain at two or three locations: the L2, L3, and L4 levels.

(2) Ten to 15 cm needles are used. The needles are inserted 7–10 cm from the midline.

(3) A 40–50 degree oblique view of the fluoroscope is used so that the skin entry site is directly in line with the ventrolateral

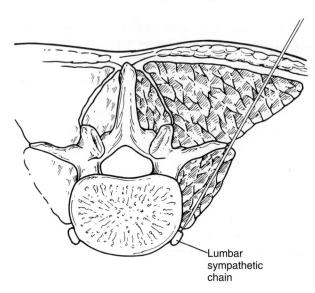

Lumbar
sympathetic
chain

Figure 3–6. Cross sectional view of the lumbar spine. The sympathetic chain and ganglion is depicted at the anterolateral aspect of the vertebral body. The path of the PRFA probe is also shown.

aspect of the vertebral body. The needle is then advanced toward the target.

(4) Many practitioners prefer to contact the transverse process first and then redirect the needle toward the vertebral body.

(5) The distance from the skin to the transverse process is roughly equal to half the distance to the vertebral body. If a 20 gauge needle is used, loss of resistance to air or saline can help identify penetration of the needle through the psoas fascia.

(6) The loss of resistance becomes unreliable with smaller gauge needles.

(7) The needle tip position should be further confirmed by injection of a water-soluble contrast agent such as iohexol.

(8) Aspiration for cerebrospinal fluid or blood should be negative, and absence of paresthesias should be confirmed.

d. Specific Complications

(1) Intravascular injection

(2) Subarachnoid injection

(3) Genitofemoral neuralgia

(4) Injury to the lumbar plexus

(5) Puncture of the renal pelvis or ureter

(6) Ejaculatory failure (bilateral block in males)

(7) Back pain

VII. Post-procedure Care

A. Patients should be observed until fully stable prior to discharge home. Thirty minutes of observation is generally adequate. Vital signs should be monitored.

B. A focused neurological examination should be documented to screen for neurological complications. For cervical and thoracic procedures, the possibility of pneumothorax should be considered.

C. For muscle spasm or soft tissue discomfort near the site of procedure, application of ice packs may be helpful.

VIII. Procedure Reporting

The following items should be included in the procedure report:

A. Informed consent

B. Patient position

C. Skin prep, sterile drape

D. Local anesthesia and sedation

E. Type of needles and RF probes used

F. Fluoroscopic or computed tomography guidance for needle placement

G. Type and amount of radiocontrast agent and description of radiographic spread

H. Neurologic stimulation, reproduction of patient's usual symptoms, paresthesias

I. PRF lesion—number of lesions and locations: temperature used; frequency and duration of process

J. Complications

IX. Procedural Coding

	CPT Code
A. Cervical medial branch PRFA	
1. Single level	64626
2. Each additional level	64627
B. Lumbar medial branch PRFA	
1. Single level	64622
2. Each additional level	64623

C. Sacral medial branch PRFA

   1. Single level   64622

   2. Each additional level   64623

D. Dorsal root ganglion (DRG) PRFA   64640

E. Stellate ganglion PRFA   64640

F. Lumbar sympathetic chain PRFA   64640

G. Thoracic sympathetic chain PRFA   64640

SUGGESTED READING

1. Bogduk N: The innervation of the lumbar spine. Spine 8:286–293, 1983.
2. Bogduk N, Long DM: Lumbar medial branch neurotomy: a modification of facet denervation. Spine 5:193–201, 1980.
3. Bogduk N, Twomey LT: Clinical anatomy of the lumbar spine. New York, Churchill Livingstone, 1987.
4. Burton CV: Percutaneous radiofrequency facet denervation. Appl Neurophysiol 39:80–86, 1977.
5. Cho J, Park YG, Chung SS: Percutaneous radiofrequency lumbar facet rhizotomy in mechanical low back pain syndrome. Stereotact Funct Neurosurg 68(1–4 Pt 1):212–217, 1997.
6. Dreyfuss, P, Halbrook B, Pauza K, et al: Efficacy and validity of radiofrequency neurotomy for chronic lumbar zygapophyseal joint pain. Spine 25(10):1270–1277, 2000.
7. Gallagher J, Vadi PLP, Wedley FR, et al: Radiofrequency facet joint denervaton in the treatment of low back pain: a prospective controlled double-blind study to assess its efficacy. The Pain Clinic 7(3):193–198, 1994.
8. Geurts JWM, Stolker RJ: Percutaneous radiofrequency lesion of the stellate ganglion in the treatment of pain in upper extremity reflex sympathetic dystrophy. The Pain Clinic 6:17–25, 1993.
9. Hayneswoth RF, Noe CE: Percutaneous lumbar sympathectomy: a comparison of radiofrequency denervation versus phenol neurolysis. Anaesthesiology 74:459–463, 1991.
10. Ketroser DB: Whiplash, chronic neck pain, and zygapophyseal joint disorders. A selective review. Minn Med 83(2):51–54, 2000.
11. Van Kleef M, Spaans F, Dingemans W, et al: Effects and side effects of a percutaneous thermal lesion of the dorsal root ganglion in patients with cervical pain syndrome. Pain 52:49–53, 1993.
12. Koning JM, Mackie DP: Percutaneous radiofrequency facet denervation in low back pain. The Pain Clinic 7:199–204, 1994.
13. Lord SM, Barnsle, L, Wallis BJ, et al: Percutaneous radiofrequency neurotomy for chronic cervical zygapophyseal-joint pain. N Engl J Med 335:1721–1726, 1996.
14. McDonald GJ, Lord SM, Bogduk N: Long-term follow-up of patients treated with cervical radiofrequency neurotomy for chronic neck pain. Neurosurgery 45:61–67, 1999.
15. Munglani R: The longer term effect of pulsed radiofrequency for neuropathic pain. Pain 80:437–439, 1999.
16. Nash TP: Percutaneous radiofrequency lesioning of dorsal root ganglia for intractable pain. Pain 24:67–73, 1986.
17. Noe CE, Haynesworth RF: Lumbar radiofrequency sympatholysis. J Vasc Surg 17:801–806, 1993.
18. North RB, Kidd DH, Campbell JN, Long DM: Dorsal root ganglionectomy for failed back surgery syndrome: A 5 year follow-up study. J Neurosurg 74:236–242, 1991.
19. Pernak J: Percutaneous radiofrequency thermal lumbar sympathectomy. The Pain Clinic 8:99–106, 1995.
20. Ray CD: Percutaneous radiofrequency facet nerve block (Radionics Procedure Technique Series). Burlington, MA, Radionics Corp, 1982.

21. Schwarzer AC, Aprill CN, Bogduk N: The sacroiliac joint in chronic low back pain. Spine 20:31–37, 1995.
22. Slappendel R, Crul BJ, Braak GJ, et al: The efficacy of radiofrequency lesioning of the cervical spinal dorsal root ganglion in a double-blinded randomized study: no difference between 40 degrees C and 67 degrees C treatments. Pain 73:159–163, 1997.
23. Sluijter ME: Radiofrequency lesions in the treatment of cervical pain syndromes (Radionics Procedure Technique Series). Burlington, MA, Radionics, 1990.
24. van Kleef M, Barendse GA, Kessels A, et al: Randomized trial of radiofrequency lumbar facet denervation for chronic low back pain. Spine 24:1937–1942, 1999.
25. van Suijlekom HA, van Kleef M, Barendse GA, et al: Radiofrequency cervical zygapophyseal joint neurotomy for cervicogenic headache: a prospective study of 15 patients. Funct Neurol 13:297–303, 1998.
26. van Kleef M, Barendse G, Dingemans W, et al: Effects of producing a radiofrequency lesion adjacent to the dorsal root ganglion in patients with thoracic segmental pain. Clin J Pain 11:325–332, 1995.
27. Wilkinson HA: Radiofrequency percutaneous upper thoracic sympathectomy. N Engl J Med 311:34–36, 1984.
28. Wilkinson HA: Radiofrequency percutaneous upper thoracic sympathectomy: a new technique. Neurosurgery 15:811–814, 1984.
29. Yarzebski JL, Wilkinson HA: T2 and T3 sympathetic ganglia in the adult human: a cadaver and clinical radiologic study and its clinical application. Neurosurgery 21:339–341, 1987.

4

Spinal Facet and Sacroiliac Joint Blocks

Robert H. Dorwart, M.D.

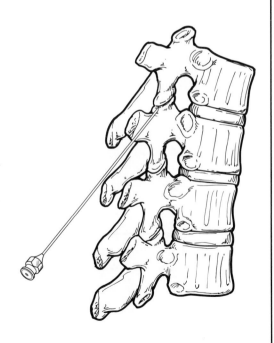

I.   Rationale

A. Spinal facet syndrome is defined variably in the medical literature. In essence, it is a condition related to inflammation of facet joints resulting in pain, usually dorsal, overlying the affected joint(s).

1. This pain can be sporadic or nearly constant, with various descriptions, including aching, stabbing, burning, gripping, and toothache-like. However, because of the innervation of spinal facet joints by the medial branch of the dorsal rami of spinal nerves, there can be associated referred pain distal to the facet.

2. At upper cervical level C2–3, pain is referred to the occipital region. At other cervical levels, pain is referred along the dorsolateral neck toward the shoulder (Fig. 4–1).

3. In the thoracic region, pain can be referred along the ipsilateral costal and intercostal region, usually only as far as the posterior axillary line (Fig. 4–2).

4. Upper lumbar facets L1–2 and L2–3 refer to the posterolateral low back and flank (Fig. 4–3), rarely to the anterolateral lower abdomen and groin.

5. The L3–4 and L4–5 facet joints refer to the ipsilateral iliac crest, buttock, hip, and upper aspect anterior thigh (Fig. 4–4).

6. The L4–5 facet sometimes refers as low as the knee, and occasionally into the anterior calf.

7. The L5–S1 facet joint refers to the buttock, posterior and lateral aspects of the thigh (sometimes as low as the knee) (Fig. 4–5), and occasionally into the lateral calf. (Bilateral referred symptoms are theoretically possible because of the cross-innervation that has been observed on microanatomic dissections, but this topic is beyond the scope of the chapter.)

8. Furthermore, the multifidus muscles attach to the posterior margins of the facet capsules, and the inflammation of facets can also affect the multifidus muscles, resulting in spasms, or "catching" sensations.

9. Facet syndrome is often associated with internal derangement of intervertebral discs and instability, which can result in actual tearing and detachment of multifidus muscles from the facet margins.

10. Clinical presentations are variable, and establishing the diagnosis can be challenging.

11. Intra-articular injections of local anesthetic solutions, as well as blocks of dorsal branches of same-level or adjacent-level spinal nerves (Fig. 4–6), can provide diagnostic information regarding the source of a patient's back or neck pain.

Text continued on page 68

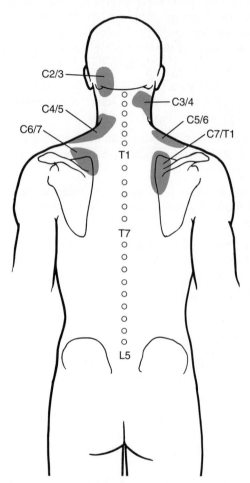

Figure 4–1. Cervical facet pain referral patterns reported by patients. (From Bogduk N, Marsland A: The cervical zygapophyseal joints as a source of neck pain. Spine 13:610–617, 1988.)

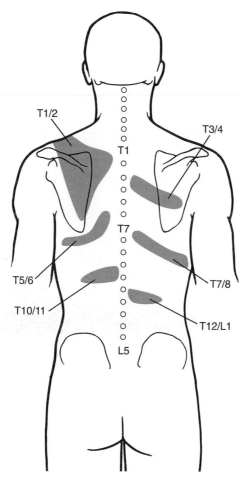

Figure 4–2. Pain referral patterns from thoracic facet joints. (From Fukui S, Ohseto K, Shiotani M: Patterns of pain induced by distending the thoracic zygapophyseal joints. Reg Anesth 22(4):332–336, 1997.)

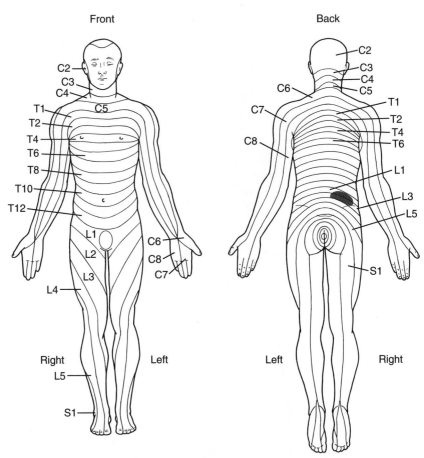

Figure 4–3. Pain drawing by a patient with right upper lumbar facet joint–induced pain. L1–2 and L2–3 facets typically refer from near the midline high lumbar area toward the flank.

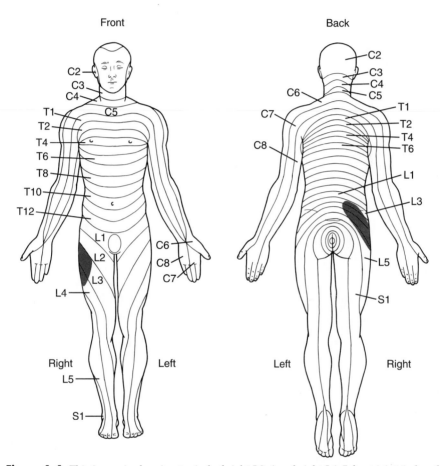

Figure 4–4. This is a pain drawing typical of right L3–4 and right L4–5 facet joint–induced pain, radiating to the iliac crest area around to the anterolateral hip and upper aspect of anterolateral thigh.

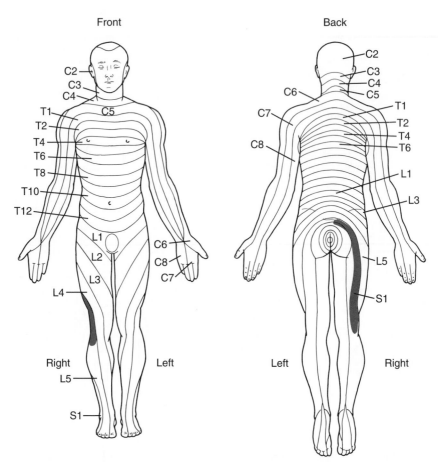

Figure 4–5. Pain drawing typical for right L5-S1 facet joint referred pain, showing pain referred through the buttock along the posterior thigh into the posterolateral knee region.

12. Concomitant injection of glucocorticoids can reduce inflammation in the joint(s), neural innervation, and paraspinal muscle attachments, providing the patient with symptomatic improvement of variable and unpredictable duration.

13. Cryoablation or radiofrequency ablative procedures provide longer-term denervation and pain relief.

B. The paired sacroiliac joints form the attachment of the spinal column to the pelvic girdle. There are synovial (diarthrodial) and fibrous components to the sacroiliac joints (Fig. 4–7). The joint capsule and ligamentous structure is complex, and various muscle origins and insertions upon the sacroiliac joint margins can result in regional and referred pain and possibly muscle spasms when the joints are inflamed.

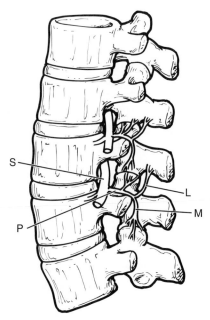

Figure 4–6. Diagrammatic representation of lumbar facet joint innervation. The spinal nerve (S) gives rise to posterior primary ramus (P). The lateral branch (L) of posterior primary ramus supplies same level facet, and the medial branch (M) has recurrent branches to the same level facet and also supplies the facet joint one level caudal to the spinal nerve of origin. (From Carrera GF, Williams AL: Current concepts in evaluation of the lumbar facet joints. CRC Crit Rev Diagn Imaging 21(2):85–104, 1985.)

1. Joint innervation is from multiple levels of spinal nerves (including medial branches of dorsal rami L5 and S1, and possibly L4, as in Fig. 4–8).
2. The sciatic nerve courses anterior to the inferior aspect of the joint, which is another potential source of referred pain patterns.
3. Intra-articular injections of anesthetic solutions, such as Marcaine or lidocaine, can provide diagnostic information, and concomitant injections of glucocorticoids can reduce joint inflammation, providing temporary reduction in pain associated with sacroiliac joint inflammation.

II.   Contraindications

A. Absolute:
1. Major hypersensitivity to anesthetic solutions or glucocorticoids
2. Local infection at the site of the proposed injection
3. Active infectious process elsewhere, including tuberculosis, because glucocorticoids suppress immunity

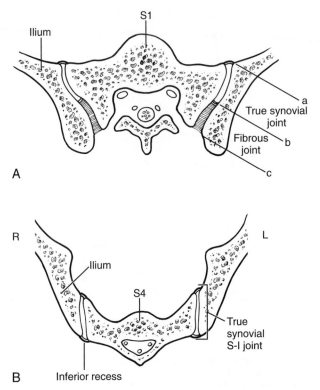

Figure 4–7. *A,* Cross-sectional representation of the sacroiliac joints at the S1 level demonstrates true synovial and fibrous components of the S-I joint at this level. *B,* Cross-sectional representation of sacroiliac joints at a more inferior S4 level demonstrates only a true synovial joint structure. At this level, the posterior joint margin is the most superficial part of the sacroiliac joint, relative to the dorsal skin surface. Thus, this is the site of easiest access to the joint. Note the inferior recess, which can serve as an indicator of successful intra-articular needle placement when it opacifies.

4. Bleeding disorders

5. Clinical disorders that contraindicate glucocorticoid therapy; e.g., actively bleeding gastric and/or duodenal ulcers, treatment-resistant diabetes mellitus, severe hypertension, and severe congestive heart failure with fluid retention

B. Relative:

1. Major hypersensitivity to iodinated contrast agents

   a. Procedure can be performed without contrast

   b. Needle position can be confirmed with spot radiographs (see section VII. Procedure)

2. Anticoagulant therapy: should be discontinued temporarily (see section VII. Procedure)

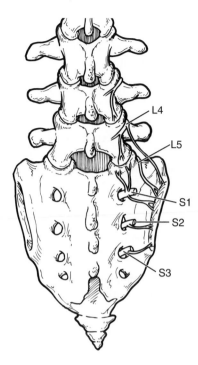

Figure 4–8. Posterior view of sacroiliac joint innervation from medial branches of dorsal rami from spinal nerves L4, L5, S1–3. (From Paris SV: Anatomy as related to function and pain. Orthop Clin North Am 14(3):475–489, 1983.)

III.   Informed Consent

A. Informed consent should be obtained from all patients. There are small but real risks such as infection and bleeding.

B. Side effects:

1. Temporary anesthesia, regional and referred, secondary to anesthetic effect

2. Insomnia for one or two nights after procedure

3. Facial flushing and acneiform facial and/or truncal rash

4. Low-grade fever 1–3 days post-procedure

5. Heartburn, stomach pain, and nausea for 1–2 days post-procedure

6. Mild-to-moderate headache secondary to glucocorticoid side effects

IV.   Pertinent Anatomy

A. All spinal facets are true synovial (diarthrodial) joints with facet capsule, articular cartilage, and a thin layer of synovium.

1. Joint bony components are the inferior articulating process from the rostral spinal segment and the superior articulating process from the caudal spinal segment.
2. Proprioceptive fibers and pain fibers innervate the facet capsule and possibly the synovium.
3. Multifidus muscles insert upon the posterior facet capsule.
4. Innervation is from small neural twigs arising from the medial and lateral branches of the dorsal ramus of the spinal nerve, which exits from the foramen corresponding to the facet level, *and* variably from the spinal nerve one level above and one level below (see Fig. 4–8).
5. Cross-innervation from the same-level opposite side spinal nerve has been observed on some microanatomic studies.

B. Plane of facet joints:
1. Cervical—oblique coronal, most easily accessed at the inferolateral margin via a straight lateral approach with the patient in decubitus position (Fig. 4–9)
2. Thoracic—oblique coronal (nearly coronal), accessible from an insertion point on the skin two facet levels caudal to the affected level to be injected, angling the needle craniad, with the patient prone (Fig. 4–10)
3. Lumbar—oblique sagittal, usually accessible from the posterolateral

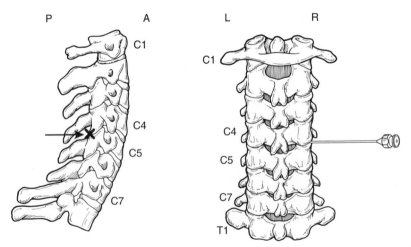

Figure 4–9. On the lateral view of cervical spine on left, ✕ marks the target point for needle insertion into the posterior margin of the C4–5 facet joint. The patient is positioned in lateral decubitus position, with left side down. PA view of the cervical spine (on the right) shows the needle course into the right C4–5 facet joint. *Note*: 25-gauge needles are best because joint spaces are small.

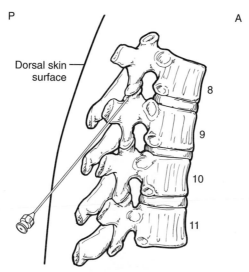

Figure 4–10. Lateral view of the thoracic spine demonstrates the needle course for the T8–9 facet joint. The patient is positioned prone. Because of the near-coronal plane of thoracic facet joints, needle insertion must be on the dorsal skin surface approximately 1½–3 levels below the target joint to allow a steep enough approach angle to enable insertion into the caudalmost margin of the joint. *Note:* The greater the thickness of the dorsal soft tissues, the more caudal must be the skin puncture site; 25-gauge needles are best because joint spaces are small.

approach with the patient prone or slightly oblique from the prone position (Fig. 4–11); *articular processes have curved surfaces, or osteophytes or accessory capsular ossicles blocking access* (Fig. 4–12)

4. Sacroiliac joints angle lateral to medial, anterior to posterior; easily accessible at the inferior joint margin that is closest to dorsal skin surface, with the patient in prone position; *articular surfaces are often curved* (Fig. 4–13)

V. Equipment and Supplies

A. Fluoroscopy unit: C-arm fluoroscopy is ideal, with x-ray-penetrable cantilevered table to allow flexibility in patient positioning and viewing from any angle. This enables visualization of the plane of the joint space along which the needle is passed with intermittent fluoroscopic checks to monitor the course of the needle into the joint.

1. The C-arm can be rapidly rotated to frontal and lateral views to confirm needle position.

2. Spot radiographic capability is essential. Digital radiography is desirable.

3. The focal spot of the x-ray tube should be 0.3 mm to optimize resolution. Coning capability is required.

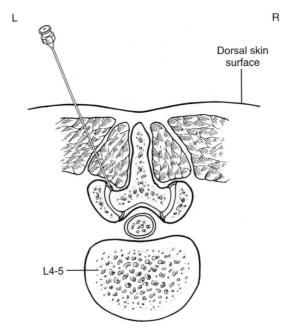

Figure 4–11. Cross-sectional depiction of the approach for lumbar facet joint needle insertion; 25-gauge or 22-gauge needles can be used. *Note:* The greater the thickness of the dorsal soft tissues, the more lateral must be the skin puncture site. Align the C-arm fluoroscopic beam along the plane of the facet joint space (along the line of the needle in this illustration).

Figure 4–12. *A,* Cross-sectional illustration of the curved lumbar facet joint anatomical variant. With this type of joint, it can be difficult to align the fluoroscopic beam with the dorsal facet opening. As the C-arm beam is rotated around a curved joint, the joint space will be visible through many degrees of rotation. Pre-procedure knowledge of this anatomy is crucial in avoiding prolonged procedures with multiple needle passages and the encountering of bone at what seems to be the joint opening (see Part 12B). Note the posterior facet capsule accessory ossicle on the right. These are usually invisible on fluoroscopic images, and such accessory bones can obstruct access. *B,* Cross-sectional illustration of potential difficulties encountered when the needle is placed into a curved lumbar facet joint space, with the patient in prone position. Needle A is aligned along the typical posterolateral approach for most lumbar facet joint punctures, but because the facet joint space is curved, the superior articulating process of L5 is encountered. Needle B is properly aligned but in a near-vertical plane that might actually result in fluoroscopic nonvisualization of the joint space. Needle C is properly aligned, but there is a posterior osteophyte blocking access to the joint. These types of difficulties can be avoided only if cross-sectional images such as CT or MRI scans are reviewed prior to performing the procedure.

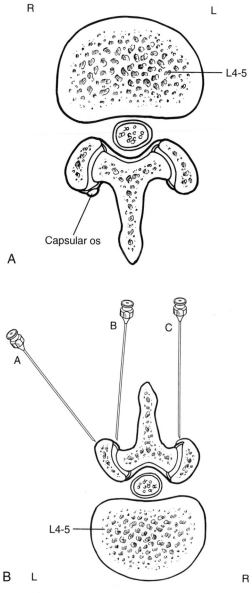

Figure 4–12. *See legend on opposite page*

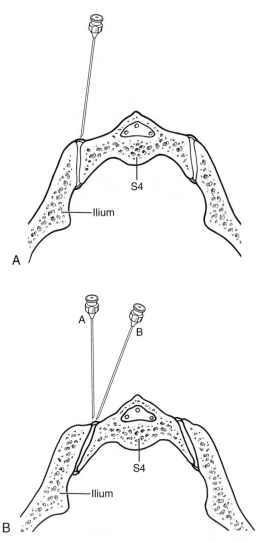

Figure 4–13. *A,* "Good" sacroiliac joint, with relatively straight joint space. The patient is positioned prone for sacroiliac needle placement, the level of the caudalmost joint is determined fluoroscopically, and with near-vertical fluoroscopic beam a 25-gauge needle is inserted, so quickly that the proceduralist may begin to think that he or she has remarkable skill. *B,* "Bad" sacroiliac joint, with multiplanar curvature and overhanging margin of ilium. The real posterior joint margin will not be visible fluoroscopically. Needle A seems to be properly aligned but the posterior ilium is encountered, and the proceduralist develops an inferiority complex. Needle B is aligned so that access to the joint with a 25-gauge needle is possible, but review of cross-sectional images such as CT or MRI is essential to avoid this pitfall.

B. CT-guided facet injection may be considered as an acceptable alternative.

C. A ceiling-mounted transparent leaded shield should be present to protect the operator. A floor-mounted lead shield with viewing window protects the x-ray technologist. The radiologist and assisting technologists should wear shielded aprons and thyroid shields. Leaded-glass eyeglasses can be used by the radiologist, if desired. The radiologist and technologist should wear exposure-monitoring badges.

D. Standard sterile tray with:

1. Two plastic trays, one for iodine-based preparation solution and one for alcohol wash

2. 4 × 4 gauze pads

3. 3, 5 or 10 ml syringes

4. 25-gauge 1½ inch needle for skin anesthesia

5. 18-gauge 1½ inch needle for aspirating solutions from vials

E. Usual needle sizes for intra-articular insertions (by region):

1. Cervical—25-gauge 2–2½ inch most common; longest needle in large and/or obese patients up to 3½–5 inches

2. Thoracic—25-gauge 3½ inch most common; in large and/or obese patients up to 5–6 inches

3. Lumbar—25-gauge (preferred) or 22-gauge (largest necessary), 3½–5 inches most common; in obese and/or large patients up to 6–7 inches (22 gauge)

4. Sacroiliac—25-gauge (22 gauge will not enter many sacroiliac joint spaces), 2–3½ inches

F. Sterile latex gloves are routinely used, with sterile thin-leaded gloves beneath the sterile latex gloves (optional for protection of the operator from radiation exposure to the hands). Reuse the leaded gloves; they are expensive! *Sterile nonlatex gloves should be available for patients with known anaphylactic reactions to latex.* Powder should be washed from gloves with alcohol.

G. Medications needed:

1. Lidocaine—1% for skin and subcutaneous anesthesia

2. Buffer solution (sodium bicarbonate 4.2%) for adding to lidocaine—1% (reduces stinging sensation)

3. Marcaine—0.5% for intra-articular and branch nerve blocks

4. Steroid medications:

a. Celestone Soluspan (6 mg betamethasone per ml, water-soluble)

   b. Depo-Medrol (20 mg, 40 mg, and 80 mg methylprednisolone per
   ml solutions are available; 40 mg/ml solution is most often used)

H. Contrast agents:

   1. Spinal facets—nonionic, water-soluble iodinated contrast agents,
   such as iopamidol and iohexol, in concentrations 180–240 mgI/ml
   are required because these injections are near the spinal canal and
   thecal sac. The higher concentration is preferred for better visualization of these small joints, especially in obese patients.

   2. Sacroiliac joints—ionic (e.g., Conray 43, etc.) or nonionic water-
   soluble iodinated contrast agents, 180–240 mg/ml (see section
   G. 1). Because toxicity and allergic reactions are less frequent, nonionic contrast agents are preferred (occasionally vascular opacification occurs with test injections for confirming needle position).
   Although the nonionic contrast is more expensive, the amounts
   used are small (3–5 ml).

VI.   Conscious Sedation

Rarely needed, but if the patient is anxious enough to require conscious
sedation, the following are options (*only one option should be used per patient*):

A. Oral liquid Valium: Total dose of 2.5–10.0 mg in partial doses of 2.5–5.0
   mg, with 10–15 minute intervals between partial doses

B. Sublingual Versed: Total dose of 0.5–2.0 mg in partial doses of 0.5 mg,
   with 10–15 minute intervals between partial doses

C. Intravenous Versed: Total dose of 0.5–2.0 mg in partial doses of 0.5 mg,
   with 5–10 minute intervals between partial doses

D. Intravenous Valium: Total dose of 2.5–10 mg in partial doses of 2.5 mg,
   with 5–10 minute intervals between partial doses

E. Baseline vital signs should be obtained prior to conscious sedation.
   Patients should be monitored with pulse oximeter; oxygen saturation
   should be maintained at 90% or greater, with supplemental oxygen by
   nasal prongs or mask at 2–4 liters/minute, if needed. Care should be
   taken when administering supplemental oxygen to patients with
   chronic obstructive pulmonary disease.

VII.   Procedure

A. Imaging studies of the region of interest should be reviewed. It should
   be remembered that some facet joints have curved joint spaces, especially lumbar levels L3–4 and L4–5 (see Fig. 4–12). This also applies to
   sacroiliac joints, which usually are curved (see Fig. 4–13).

   1. At fluoroscopy, the plane of the posterior margin of the facet or

sacroiliac joint can be difficult or impossible to visualize. Instead, the more anterior joint space plane may be visualized, resulting in an erroneous approach angle.

2. In addition, facet and sacroiliac joints might have hypertrophic spurs at their posterior margins, which can block access to the joint space.

3. It might be necessary to approach a facet joint at its cranial or caudal margin, or at a point anywhere between these, to find a pathway into the joint.

4. Taking these anatomic and pathologic features into account before the procedure can save much time.

B. Facet levels to be injected should be correlated with a pain drawing, which the patient completes prior to the procedure (as in Figs. 4–3 through 4–5).

1. This is helpful in determining appropriate facet levels to be injected and to help determine whether medial branch nerve block should be undertaken (if there is referred pain).

2. In addition, the baseline pre-procedure drawing can be correlated with the post-procedure drawing to ascertain response to the injected anesthetic.

C. *An informed consent form should be signed prior to conscious sedation,* if such is to be given. Mention of the risk of bleeding and infection should be included.

1. Patients should be warned of temporary anesthesia in the region of injection and possibly referred anesthesia distal to the injection site.

2. They should be instructed regarding glucocorticoid side effects (see section III. B2.)

3. A brief clinical history of pertinent conditions relative to steroid effects should be obtained, such as active infection including tuberculosis, gastric and/or duodenal ulcers, hypertension, and advanced congestive heart failure.

4. An allergic history should be obtained.

D. Conscious sedation can be administered at this point, if necessary. *It is rarely required if these procedures are properly and carefully performed.*

1. The proceduralist should approach the patient in a calm, confident manner. Casual conversation with the patient during the procedure is very helpful in establishing rapport and helps to distract the patient. Ask patients where they live, what their occupation is, and what their hobbies and interests are.

2. Often these conversations are very interesting and insight can be

gained into patients' psychological status and understanding (or lack thereof) of their disease.

E. Positioning

1. *Cervical facet*: The plane of joint space is oblique from true coronal. The caudal and lateral margin of the joint is most easily accessed (see Fig. 4–9). The patient is positioned decubitus with the *side of interest up*. The level is localized with lateral fluoroscopy, counting down from C2, which is easily recognized. The skin is marked using an opaque device such as a ballpoint pen tip touching the patient's skin at projected needle entry site, then marked with a felt-tip marker such as a Sharpie.

2. *Thoracic facet*: The plane of joint is slightly oblique from true coronal. Use of the lateral approach such as in the cervical region is unfeasible because of the width of the trunk. The patient is prone with level of interest localized, which might be challenging in the thoracic region. The number of rib-bearing thoracic segments should be confirmed either fluoroscopically or with scout AP radiograph of thoracic region pre-procedure. Counting can be either from the first or last rib. A parasagittal plane along the line of the articular processes ipsilateral to the facet to be injected is selected and the skin is marked as discussed in section E. 1, 1½–3 levels caudal to the facet joint to be injected. This is necessary because of the steep near-coronal plane of the thoracic facet joints (see Fig. 4–10). Some authors advocate performing medial branch nerve blocks in lieu of thoracic intra-articular facet injections because of the difficulty in approaching the thoracic facet joints.[12] For this technique, see section E. 5 (below).

3. *Lumbar facet*: The plane of these joints is usually oblique from the true sagittal plane. The patient is positioned prone, or slightly prone oblique, if necessary for patient comfort. Localize lumbar facets by counting upward from the S1 segment. Determine the plane of joint space by observing fluoroscopically as the C-arm is rotated slowly about the axial plane of the joint to be injected (see Fig. 4–11). Mark the skin as discussed in E. 1. *Remember: L3–4 and L4–5 facets might have a curved joint space* (see Fig. 4–12). Review of previous cross-sectional imaging studies is ideal preparation for selecting the best approach angle. CT-guided needle insertion is rarely necessary. The CT-guided technique is more cumbersome, because localization of the skin insertion point is awkward and needle advancement is "blind" (relative to intermittent and multiplanar imaging provided by the real-time fluoroscopic approach).

4. *Sacroiliac joint*: The plane of these joints is usually oblique from true sagittal and the articular surfaces are usually curved (see Fig. 4–13).

The joint is most easily accessed at its caudalmost margin, where the anterior-posterior dimension of the joint is short. Thus, there is less likely to be confusion as to which aspect of the joint space is tangent to the fluoroscopic beam, so *the fluoroscopic beam should be centered over the caudal aspect of the sacroiliac joint.* Usually, the correct plane of the beam is vertical or nearly vertical, with the patient prone. Determine the plane of the caudalmost sacroiliac joint and mark the overlying skin as discussed in E. 1.

5. *Nerve blocks of medial branches of dorsal rami*: These injections are primarily diagnostic procedures that might be performed if the patient reports a pain syndrome with referred pain that is a major component of his or her complaints (25% or more of the pain syndrome accompanying pain localized to the affected facet). Medial branch blocks should be performed on the level(s) most likely to be responsible for the referred component of the patient's pain; *thus, use of pain drawings by the patient and knowledge of usual referred pain patterns are essential for determination of appropriate injections to be made.* Needle positions for these injections are close to those used for the intra-articular facet injections. The same needle used for a facet injection can be repositioned into the appropriate medial branch location(s) (Figs. 4–14 to 4–16), and 1.0–1.5 ml of Marcaine 0.5% *or* lidocaine 2% can be injected.

F. Skin preparation and local anesthetic

1. Wash the skin overlying the region of interest at least twice with an iodine cleansing solution such as betadine, over an area at least 20 cm^2 surrounding the needle insertion point.

2. Have alcohol wash available in a second sterile plastic basin. Use this to wash powder from gloves at the onset of the procedure. Use the solution intermittently throughout the procedure to maintain glove sterility by dipping fingers in the alcohol wash.

3. Anesthetize the skin and underlying subcutaneous tissues with buffered lidocaine 1%. *Note*: Buffering the lidocaine with sodium bicarbonate 4.2%, available in 5 ml vials, reduces skin stinging. A 2:1 lidocaine:buffer is employed (e.g., 3 ml lidocaine 1% and 1.5 ml sodium bicarbonate 4.2%).

G. Needle insertion and injection of intra-articular contrast

1. Needle insertion is performed with *gentle, small incremental advances* while observing fluoroscopically intermittently. Occasional use of orthogonal plane fluoroscopic views will help the proceduralist maintain three-dimensional orientation.

2. *Confirmatory spot radiographs* should be obtained AP, lateral, and oblique after intra-articular contrast is observed fluoroscopically, *prior to* injecting anesthetic/glucocorticoid solution.

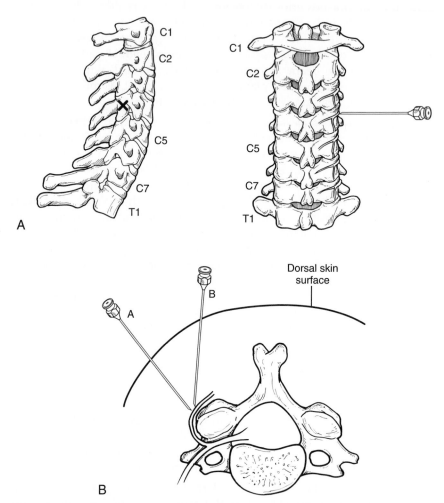

Figure 4–14. *A*, Lateral view (*left*) and PA (*right*) views of needle placement for cervical medial branch nerve blocks. The patient is positioned lateral decubitus with the *side of interest up* for cervical facet joint injection (C4–5 for this illustration; also see Figure 4–9). The needle is removed from the facet joint and is repositioned to the lateral margin of the articular column of the same level, where 1.0–1.5 cc of either Marcaine 0.5% or lidocaine 2% is injected for diagnostic medial branch nerve block. Also see part *B*. (From Bogduk N: Back pain: Zygapophyseal blocks and epidural steroids. In Cousins M, Bridenbaugh PO (eds): Neural Blockade in Clinical Anesthesia and Management of Pain, Second Edition. Philadelphia, J.B. Lippincott, 1988, pp 935–946.) *B*, Cross-sectional illustration of optional approaches for cervical medial branch blocks. Near-vertical (*A*) or posterolateral oblique (*B*) approaches with the patient positioned prone can be utilized. Also see part *A*. (From McDonald GJ, Lord SM, Bogduk N: Long-term follow-up of patients treated with cervical radiofrequency neurotomy for chronic neck pain. *Neurosurgery* 45(1):61–68, 1999.)

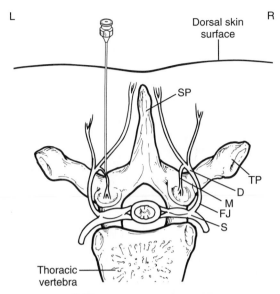

Figure 4–15. Cross-sectional illustration of near-vertical needle course and placement for thoracic medial branch block. The patient is positioned prone, the appropriate level is localized by counting the total number of rib-bearing thoracic segments. Injection of 1.0–1.5 cc Marcaine 0.5% or lidocaine 2% is performed after careful determination of the location of the needle tip with PA and lateral fluoroscopic and digital radiographic images. SP = spinous process, TP = right transverse process, FJ = right facet joint, S = right thoracic spinal nerve, D = dorsal ramus, M = medial branch. (From Waldman SD: Thoracic facet block: medial branch technique. In *Atlas of Interventional Pain Management*. Philadelphia, W.B. Saunders Co., 1998, pp 216–219.)

3. As much iodinated contrast solution should be aspirated as possible prior to injection of anesthetic/glucocorticoid solution. (Often no contrast can be aspirated. Don't worry—press on!)

H. Injection of anesthetic/glucocorticoid solutions:

1. Mix Marcaine 0.5% *or* lidocaine 2% with glucocorticoid solution (*either* Celestone Soluspan *or* Depo-Medrol) in 1 ml:1 ml admixture

2. Usual intra-articular volumes of mixed injectate:

   a. Cervical and thoracic facet joints—0.5–0.75 ml

   b. Lumbar facet joints—1.0–2.0 ml

   c. Sacroiliac joints—2.0–3.0 ml

   Note: Use 3 ml or 5 ml syringes to ensure adequate injection pressure.

3. When multiple joint injections are to be made, total glucocorticoid volumes should be limited to:

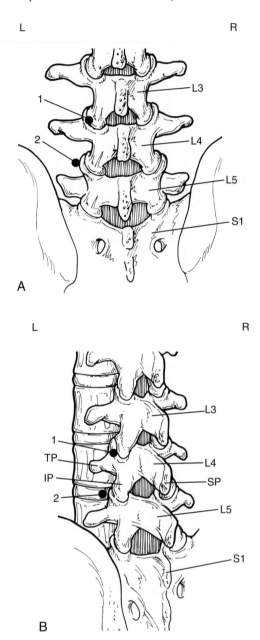

Figure 4-16. *A,* Lumbar medial branch blocks require upper (1) and lower (2) targets, since they innervate the nearest joint and the joint one level rostral to the spinal nerve of origin. Targets 1 and 2 should be injected with 1.0–1.5 cc Marcaine 0.5% or lidocaine 2% for left L4 medial branch block, in this illustration. The patient is positioned prone, and oblique postero-lateral needle course is employed. *B,* Illustration of posterolateral oblique view of upper and lower target points for L4 medial branch block. TP = transverse process L4, SP = spinous process L4, IP = inferior articulating process L4, IC = iliac crest. (A and B From Dreyfuss P, Schwarzer AC, Lau P et al: Specificity of lumbar medial branch and 1% dorsal ramus blocks. *Spine* 22(8):895–902, 1997.)

a. Celestone Soluspan 2.5 ml for an average adult, up to 3.0 ml for large patients, *or*

b. Depo-Medrol 80–100 mg for an average adult, up to 120 mg for large patients

Higher doses result in more severe side effects.

I. During the procedure, the patient experiences:

1. Local jab from the anesthetic needle

2. 2–3 seconds of burning sensation from skin anesthesia

3. Intermittent pressure sensations during needle insertion

4. Possible localized pain sensation when the needle passes through the joint capsule

5. Pressure during injection of medications, especially near the end of the injection when the joint is near capacity

J. After the procedure, the patient can anticipate localized anesthesia at the injection site and possibly referred along the course of the usual pain (if the patient had referred pain symptoms) and, hopefully, partial or complete (but temporary) relief of pain. The initial pain reduction is related to local anesthetic effects and may last 30–60 minutes if lidocaine 2% is injected into the joint or 1–4 hours if Marcaine 0.5% is used. The therapeutic effects of glucocorticoids are usually noticed after a 1–2 day delay, and the condition will gradually improve over 3–7 days post-procedure. The duration of effect is variable from brief (1–7 days) to longer, as long as several weeks to several months, depending on the success of glucocorticoid suppression of joint and neural inflammation and also depending on the underlying pathology and subsequent therapy.

K. Should injections be repeated? Some practitioners advocate routine use of a series of three injections; others recommend single injections repeated as necessary up to a total of three, with 10–14 day intervals between injections. Glucocorticoids have side effects as listed in section III. B. Glucocorticoids temporarily suppress the immune system, and as a rule of thumb, after a series of injections has been performed, there should be a 60–90 day injection-free period to allow the immune system to recover.

VIII. Post-procedure Care

A. Wash iodine scrub solution from skin, apply Band-Aid(s) over puncture site(s), and instruct the patient to leave Band-Aids in place overnight.

B. Explain expected results as discussed in J. above. A few minutes of education usually saves telephone callbacks. The patient should be informed of glucocorticoid side effects. An information and instruction

form should be given to the patient, including side effects and anticipated results and telephone callback information.

C. If the patient is stable and self-ambulatory, allow him or her to dress.
Patients must remain in waiting area 15–20 minutes after dressing, at
which time their clinical status is briefly assessed and they are asked to
report immediate results. Pre-injection pain (severity and location) is
compared to post-injection anesthesia and pain relief. Residual pain
(severity and location) can be indicated on a pain drawing. Pain severity
can be graded on a subjective 0–10 scale.

D. The patient is discharged if clinically stable. The goal is a positive
response by the patient to an uneventful procedure and partial or
complete pain relief.

IX. Reporting the Procedure

A. Patient name, date of birth, identification number, and date of procedure

B. Procedure title and examination: e.g., "Right L4–5 facet Arthrography
and Therapeutic Injection of Marcaine/Celestone." It is important to be
detailed and specific; this will facilitate records review and reimbursement approval (desired results of efforts exerted in reporting details).

C. First report section should be entitled **Procedures Performed**. This must
include a brief description of the procedure and supplies used, to assist
the reimbursement reviewer in determining appropriateness of charges
and amount to reimburse.

1. *Example A*: "Right L4–5 Facet Arthrography and Therapeutic Injection of Marcaine and Celestone"

   Procedures Performed:

   a. Injection into the facet joint and/or facet joint nerve
   b. AP, oblique, and lateral spine radiography and interpretation
   c. Use of fluoroscopy for spinal injection
   d. Noncontrast materials (gown, gloves, needles, tubing, syringes,
   and spinal tray)
   e. Use of low osmolar (nonionic) contrast
   f. Celestone Soluspan (*or* Depo-Medrol) and Marcaine
   g. Buffered lidocaine

2. *Example B*: "Right Sacroiliac Joint Arthrogram and Therapeutic Injection of Marcaine and Celestone"

   Procedures Performed:

   a. Sacroiliac joint arthrography supervision and interpretation

    b. Intra-articular injection of local anesthetic and steroid

    c. Nonionic materials (gown, gloves, needles, tubing, syringes, and spinal tray)

    d. Celestone Soluspan (*or* Depo-Medrol) and Marcaine

    e. Buffered lidocaine

D. Second section of report: **Clinical Information**. Age and sex of patient, brief pertinent clinical history that justifies the procedure, e.g., "45-year-old man with chronic right lower back and right buttock pain, worse with exercise; MRI reveals right L4–5 facet and periarticular inflammation and hypertrophic osteoarthritis."

E. Third section of report: **Technical Information**. Begin with the sentence about informed consent obtained and signed, then write a brief description of skin preparation and draping in the usual manner, buffered lidocaine 1% local anesthesia, gauge and length of the needle (helpful reference for possible future repeat injections), successful placement with fluoroscopic guidance into the joint(s), test injection of contrast (amount, type, and concentration), confirmatory spot radiographs (specify digital, if so done; specify planes taken, e.g., AP, lateral, and oblique). Specify type, concentration, and amount of local anesthetic and glucocorticoid injected into joint(s). Indicate that pre-injection pain was recorded and will be compared with post-injection pain. Report monitoring time in the clinic after the procedure. *Example:* "The procedure of facet joint arthrography and associated risks, including bleeding and infection, were discussed with the patient, who signed an informed consent form. (*If conscious sedation was used*, describe baseline vital signs, type of sedation, amount, and monitoring technique.) The skin overlying the region was prepared in the usual sterile manner and draped. Buffered lidocaine 1% skin anesthesia was employed. Under fluoroscopic guidance, a 25 gauge 3½ inch needle was inserted into the right L4–5 facet joint, and a test amount of 0.5–0.75 ml Omnipaque 240 was injected. After confirmation of intra-articular needle position, a mixture of Marcaine 0.5% and Celestone Soluspan was injected into the facet joint. The needle was removed, and the patient was monitored for 15–20 minutes after the procedure to determine clinical status and initial response to the injections. Pre-procedural pain level and distribution were compared with post-injection pain level and distribution."

F. Fourth section of report: **Interpretation and Results**. State briefly pertinent abnormalities on spot radiographs, if any, and state that spot radiographs confirmed the appropriate site of needle placement. Indicate whether the needle was intra-articular and that joint space was opacified. Indicate type, concentration, and amount of injectate into joint(s). Report results with comparison of pre-injection pain with post-injection pain. Report time in the clinic post-procedure and patient status at discharge.

G. Final section of report: **Conclusion**. This is summary statement of success of procedure and initial results, e.g., "Technically successful right L4–5 arthrogram and intra-articular therapeutic injections, with immediate relief of patient's usual right lower back and buttock pain in response to Marcaine. The therapeutic effects of the injected glucocorticoid are expected to have onset at 1–2 days post-procedure, which will be monitored in follow-up by (referring M.D.)" This last statement returns the patient to the referring physician's care.

X. Procedural Coding

A. *Cervical facet joint(s)*

	CPT Code
1. First level	64470
2. Each additional level	64472
3. X-ray cervical spine	72050
4. Fluoroscopy	76005
5. Noncontrast supplies	A4649
6. Low-osmolar contrast medium	A4645
7. Celestone Soluspan	J0702
8. Lidocaine/Marcaine	J2000

B. *Thoracic facet joint(s)*: Same as Cervical except *instead of* x-ray cervical:

	CPT Code
X-ray thoracic	72074

C. *Lumbar facet joint(s)*

	CPT Code
1. First level	64475
2. Each additional level	64476
3. X-ray lumbar spine	72110
4. Fluoroscopy	76005
5. Noncontrast supplies	A4649
6. Low-osmolar contrast medium	A4645
7. Celestone Soluspan	J0702
8. Lidocaine/Marcaine	J2000

D. *Sacroiliac joint(s)*

	CPT Code
1. Sacroiliac joint injection	27096
2. Supervision and Interpretation	73542

3. Noncontrast supplies	A4649
4. Celestone Soluspan	J0702
5. Lidocaine/Marcaine	J2000

SUGGESTED READING

1. Bogduk N, Long D: The anatomy of the so-called "articular nerves" and their relationship to facet denervation in the treatment of low back pain. J Neurosurg 51:172–177, 1979.
2. Bogduk N, Lord S: Cervical zygapophysial joint pain. Neurosurgery Quarterly 8(2):107–117, 1998.
3. Carrera GF, Williams AL: Current concepts in evaluation of the lumbar facet joints. CRC Crit Rev Diagn Imaging 21(2):85–104, 1985.
4. Cavanaugh JM, Cuneyt Ozaktay A, Yamashita T, et al: Mechanisms of low back pain. A neurophysiologic and neuroanatomic study. Clin Orthop Related Res 335:166–180, 1997.
5. Dreyfuss P, Tibiletti C, Dreyer SJ: Thoracic zygapophyseal joint pain patterns. A study in normal volunteers. Spine 19(7):807–811, 1994.
6. Falco FJE: Lumbar spine injection procedures in the management of low back pain. Occupational Medicine: State of the Art Reviews 13(1):121–149, 1998.
7. Gray DP, Bajwa ZH, Warfield CA: Facet Block and Neurolysis. In Waldman SD (ed): Interventional Pain Management. Philadelphia, W.B. Saunders Co., 2001, pp 434–445.
8. Helbig T, Lee CK: The lumbar facet syndrome. Spine 13(1):61–64, 1988.
9. Maldjian C, Mesgarzadeh M, Tehranzadeh J: Diagnostic and therapeutic features of facet and sacroiliac joint injection. Anatomy, pathophysiology, and technique. Radiol Clin North Am 1:497–508, 1998.
10. Murtagh FR: Computed tomography and fluoroscopy guided anesthesia and steroid injection in facet syndrome. Spine 13(6):686–689, 1988.
11. Simon S: Sacroiliac joint injection and low back pain. In Waldman SD (ed): Interventional Pain Management. Philadelphia, W.B. Saunders Co., 2001, pp 535–540.
12. Waldman SD. Thoracic Facet Block: Medial Branch Technique, Atlas of Interventional Pain Management. Philadelphia, W.B. Saunders Co., 1988, pp 216–219.

5

Intraspinal Cyst Aspiration

Andrew L. Wagner, M.D.
and F. Reed Murtagh, M.D.

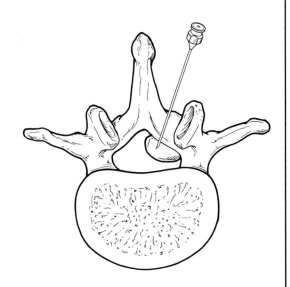

I. Rationale for Procedures and Clinical Indications

A. Cystic lesions within the spinal axis lend themselves well to ameliora-
tion by image-guided drainage techniques, but they are not all of the
same origin.

   1. Nerve root sheath cysts are filled with CSF that presumably has
entered through a one-way valve mechanism and cannot get out; the
cysts gradually enlarge and may cause root compression, potentially
relieved by needle drainage techniques such as those described in
this chapter. When nerve root sheath cysts are associated with sacral
nerve roots, they may cause bone erosion and the resulting complex
can be legitimately termed a Tarlov cyst. Tarlov cyst refers not only
to the cyst itself, lined by arachnoid, but also to the resulting eroded
sacral defect it produces.

   2. An "arachnoid cyst" is the same as a "subarachnoid cyst" and refers
to a walled-off arachnoid lined pouch with a ball valve mechanism
that gradually may enlarge and act like an intradural, extra-axial
mass within the spinal canal. "Arachnoid cyst" will be used throughout this text, arbitrarily, for consistency.

   3. A "synovial cyst" is an entirely different entity, although it may
produce symptoms of neural compression just like an arachnoid cyst
and can also be located within the spinal canal. It is synovial lined,
contains synovial fluid instead of CSF, and typically arises from a
facet joint in the dorsolateral spinal canal. It may produce an
extradural mass effect on neural structures. The synovial cyst wall
may calcify; however, synovial cysts are potentially amenable to
needle drainage using image-guided techniques described in this
chapter.

   4. Although these varied cystic lesions have different etiologies as
noted above and in the test to follow, the decision was made to
include them all together in one chapter because of the similarities
of therapeutic approach.

B. Nerve root sheath cysts are benign arachnoid-lined collections of cerebrospinal fluid that arise in the nerve root axilla at the exit foramen;
they can occur at any level of the spine. Most often seen associated
with lumbar nerve roots, they are rarely symptomatic, except if they
occur along one or more of the sacral nerves where they can be collec-
tively and rather loosely referred to as Tarlov cysts.

C. Tarlov cysts are benign perineural cysts first described by Tarlov in
1938 as incidental findings on autopsy. They are found in approximately
5% to 14% of the population,[1-3] almost always involving the sacral
nerve roots, particularly S2 and S3.

1. These cysts can rarely cause symptoms ranging from back pain and sciatica to urinary incontinence, penile or vaginal parasthesias, and lower extremity paresis.[4, 5]

2. The problem encountered by radiologists and neurosurgeons lies in differentiating symptomatic Tarlov cysts from incidental cysts in patients whose complaints originate from other spinal pathology.

3. Theoretically, these cysts have in common an ostium that communicates with the rest of the subarachnoid space via a one-way ball valve mechanism that allows filling during normal transmitted systolic CSF pulsatility but disallows subsequent emptying during diastole.

D. Percutaneous aspiration of nerve root sheath cysts, and particularly Tarlov cysts suspected to be the source of a patient's symptoms, is a safe, minimally invasive technique that will either confirm or disprove the cyst as the cause of the patient's complaints.

1. Patients who have their cysts drained may experience temporary symptomatic relief from 1 week to 6 months following the procedure, if the cysts are responsible.[2, 6] Symptoms will recur when the cyst re-fills.

2. If patients do achieve long-term relief, they may elect to continue with periodic drainages, but if the symptoms improve from drainage, surgical intervention may be indicated as a more permanent form of therapy.

E. Until recently, surgeons have been hesitant to operate on patients with Tarlov cysts due to the difficulty in proving that the cyst is symptomatic and lack of consensus on appropriate surgery.

1. Transection of the associated nerve root, with resultant permanent neurologic deficit along with pain relief, is the only way to ensure that the cyst does not recur.[7]

2. Percutaneous aspiration has not been shown to offer permanent relief, and percutaneous fibrin glue injection resulted in a high incidence of aseptic meningitis.[8]

F. Recent advances in microneurosurgical technique and CSF shunting have resulted in an improved resolution of sciatica and incontinence in patients with symptomatic sacral cysts.

1. Bartles advocated a trial of lumbar canal CSF drainage with permanent shunt placement if symptoms resolve.[9]

2. The same diagnostic information can be obtained by a simple aspiration of the cyst itself.

3. Mummaneni described patients with symptomatic Tarlov cysts treated with microsurgical techniques, including fat or muscle grafts and fibrin glue application.[10] Seven of eight patients in this study had at least moderate pain improvement and two out of three with urinary incontinence had relief following surgery.

4. With the advent of these novel neurosurgical techniques, patients with symptomatic relief following what amounts to a trial drainage of a Tarlov cyst may be permanently helped by surgical option.

G. The preceding information applies to percutaneous drainage of any nerve root cyst anywhere in the spine, but few outside of the sacral area have ever been implicated in causation of symptoms.

    1. Sacral (Tarlov) cysts are much more likely to produce symptoms because they may contain nerve rootlets in outer layers.

    2. Pressure enlargement of such a cyst erodes surrounding sacral bone and compresses neural elements against the remodeling sacral cortex.

    3. This creates stimulation of the compressed rootlets and is perceived as pain.

    4. Outside of the sacrum, none of the nerve root foramina have enough encasing bone to result in neural compression.

H. Arachnoid cysts may occur anywhere inside the spinal canal as a result of congenital duplications of arachnoid layers resulting in ball-valve mechanism filling of arachnoid diverticula, or as a result of scarring after inflammatory reactions, infections, or hemorrhage. They are intradural, extra-axial lesions, whereas nerve root cysts are not only extra-axial but also extraspinal in location.

 I. Arachnoid cysts most often occur in the dorsal aspect of the thoracic spine. Trial drainage is similar to that described for synovial cysts in the sections that follow.

 J. Synovial cysts are extradural lesions that are associated with degenerative osteoarthritis of the synovial-lined facet joints. They are not of arachnoidal origin and do not contain CSF.

    1. Most commonly occurring in the lumbar region, they can also occur in the thoracic and cervical spine.

    2. Degenerative osteoarthritis of the facet joints results in synovial hypertrophy, forming a synovial fluid-filled cyst that would be termed a "ganglion cyst" if it occurred in any other joint in the body outside of the spine.

    3. The synovial cyst will calcify, an example of the periarticular calcification that is a hallmark of degenerative osteoarthritis.

    4. Synovial cysts can be an intrinsic source of pain because the synovium is richly innervated with unmyelinated C fibers that carry pain sensation from an arthritic joint.

    5. Synovial cysts can also cause pain or other symptoms by compression of neural structures within the spinal canal, an acquired form of spinal stenosis.

K. If any specific synovial cyst is clinically thought to be a source of pain directly, as in a pain-generating arthritic joint, a trial of CT-guide aspiration and consideration of intra-articular steroid injection for pain relief may be indicated.

L. If the cyst is believed to be causing symptoms through a mechanism of spinal stenosis, CT aspiration to reduce the size of the cyst and thereby increase the area of the spinal canal may be indicated.

II.   Contraindications and Cautions

A. There are no absolute contraindications to percutaneous aspiration of nerve root sheath cysts, intraspinal subarachnoid cysts, or Tarlov cysts, apart from the situation of patients with obstructive hydrocephalus, in whom a CSF leak could be disastrous. There are no absolute contraindications to synovial cyst drainage.

B. Relative contraindications include coagulation abnormalities and immunocompromised status due to the remote risks of bleeding and meningitis, respectively.

C. It is important that gentle aspiration be used when any intraspinal or extraspinal arachnoid cyst is drained, because forceful aspiration may provoke severe pain and injure the associated nerve root.

D. For synovial cysts, it will not be possible to drain a cyst that is heavily calcified. Synovial fluid is also usually more viscous than CSF and therefore difficult to aspirate.

E. Drainage or injection of any of these cysts, whether of arachnoid or synovial origin, occurring in the cervical or thoracic spine, should be dealt with cautiously or deferred because of the possibility of spinal cord damage due to sudden changes of intraspinal pressure dynamics.

III.   Informed Consent

A. Informed consent should discuss the rationale for the procedure and the basic technique, whether for drainage of nerve root sheath cyst, Tarlov cyst, arachnoid cyst, or synovial cyst.

B. Risks are minimal for all types of drainages but include:
   1. Bleeding
   2. Infection of the CSF or soft tissues
   3. Injury to the associated nerve root
   4. Injury to the spinal cord in the cervical or thoracic regions, or the cauda equina in the lumbar area
   5. CSF leak; not likely with synovial cyst drainage but always a possibility

C. It is important to warn the patient that at the end of Tarlov cyst drainage procedure there may be a short, sharp pain in one or both legs or in the perineum, caused by contact of the needle with the neuronal fibers in the cyst wall or by the induced alterations of CSF dynamics and cyst wall pressure.

1. It is useful to give the patient a prepared form that discusses the procedure, risks, benefits, and alternatives in layman's terms prior to face-to-face discussion.

2. By having the patient sign such a sheet, another layer of evidence is added to the informed consent. A consent form also should be signed.

3. Encourage the patient to evaluate and further research the problem on the Internet. A fully educated patient is desired.

4. In order to prevent subsequent disappointment, it must be stressed to the patient that this is a diagnostic test to determine appropriate therapy and that any symptomatic relief will be temporary.

5. In actuality, patients with potentially symptomatic Tarlov cysts may arrive for an initial visit fully armed with Internet data and may have an excellent understanding of the disease process and the availability (or nonavailability) of therapeutic options.

D. Expected pain is minimal with any of the described interventions.

E. None of these procedures should be considered a permanent cure. Mostly, they afford temporary relief while the cyst (nerve root, arachnoid, or synovial) slowly refills and becomes recurrently symptomatic. The tests should be regarded by the patient as affording at best temporary relief and as a positive predictor of possible more permanent relief from a surgical procedure that might more effectively address the problem.

IV. Pertinent Anatomy

A. Tarlov cysts are really sacral perineural cysts that typically arise from the second or third sacral nerve roots. They may be unilateral only but often are so large as to obscure exact origin. Although nerve root sheath cysts can arise anywhere else in the spinal axis, they are most common in the sacral area and almost never are responsible for symptomatology in cervical, thoracic, or lumbar areas.

B. Tarlov cysts are classified as Nabor's Type II spinal meningeal cysts (extradural meningeal cysts with spinal nerve root fibers), because neural tissue is almost always included in the cyst wall.[11]

1. The wall itself is an extension of the arachnoid and dura of the sacral roots, and the cyst forms between the perineurium and the endoneurium.

2. Tarlov initially proposed that the cysts occurred following trauma due to hemosiderin deposition blocking the venous drainage of the perineurium and epineurium or arachnoidal scarring, resulting in the ball valve ostial deformity responsible for cyst formation.[12] The same theory may apply to the formation of spinal nerve root cysts anywhere in the spine or to any other subarachnoid cysts within the spinal canal.

3. Fortuna theorized that Tarlov cysts and all other nerve root cysts are a result of arachnoidal proliferation along the affected root.[13] Intraspinal arachnoid cysts might similarly result from arachnoidal proliferation within the subarachnoid spaces.

4. The currently accepted theory is that formation of a nerve root sheath cyst in any location is due to narrowing of the nerve root sheath at its ostium, forming the ball valve effect. This could be congenital, post-traumatic, or due to a combination of all of the factors mentioned.

5. The ostial narrowing forms a one-way valve that allows CSF into but not out of the cyst in response to normal CSF systolic and diastolic pulsations.

6. This may explain why some successful therapy involves treating the cysts with lumbar CSF shunting.

7. The CSF pulsations also result in characteristic scalloping of the posterior sacrum and enlargement of the sacral foramina in many cases, which can be seen on plain radiographs.

   a. CT will demonstrate the sacral scalloping and foraminal enlargement and will allow visualization of the cyst itself. Tarlov cysts are variable in size but will always have CSF attenuation, with no associated soft tissue mass.

   b. Classic myelographic descriptions of Tarlov cysts using oil-based contrast agents described delayed filling of the cyst. With the water-based contrast agents used today, the cysts typically fill quickly, although there are some that will not demonstrate a connection with CSF on myelography. Some cysts show delayed filling and no cysts empty readily. Contrast can be found in the cysts long after it has been absorbed from the rest of the subarachnoid space, but it will eventually be absorbed.

   c. Diagnosis is initially made with magnetic resonance (MR), which demonstrates characteristic well-corticated round or oval collections of CSF signal intensity eroding portions of the sacrum. These can achieve extremely large size and may even erode into the pelvis.

      (1) There will not be any enhancement on post-contrast imaging and the cysts are often multiple.

(2) The second and third sacral nerve roots are typically involved.

(3) MR myelography and flow-sensitive MR techniques can be used in further evaluation of sacral cysts, although the amount of additional relevant information provided is questionable.[14, 15]

(4) Differential diagnosis on MR imaging would include nerve sheath tumors and other benign spinal cysts such as arachnoid cysts and lumbar synovial cysts.

C. Nerve root sheath cysts elsewhere in the spinal axis arise at the lateral edge of the arachnoid space as the dural sleeve that accompanies the individual nerve root through the nerve root foramen becomes more intimate with the outer layer (perineurium) of the nerve root itself.

1. The dural sleeve eventually becomes the perineurium of the more peripheral nerve root; this first occurs just lateral to the nerve root foramen.

2. It is at this location the nerve root sheath cysts are most likely to occur.

D. Intraspinal arachnoid cysts usually occur in the thoracic region within the dorsal subarachnoid space. They form intradural, extra-axial masses and are not neoplastic.

E. Intraspinal arachnoid cysts are difficult to diagnose on MR imaging because they have the same signal characteristics as the CSF surrounding them in the spinal canal on all MR sequences.

F. Synovial cysts arise from the facet joints that are located in pairs dorsal to the spinal canal at all levels of the spinal axis.

1. Facet joints in each of the three regions of the spine have specialized anatomy pertinent to their relative functions on lending support to the spinal column dorsally while at the same time allowing for rotational movement in several planes.

2. Lumbar facet joints are larger, bear more weight, and undergo more torsional forces than those in the thoracic or cervical areas. They have more synovium and more joint area, and are more likely to develop degenerative osteoarthritis and synovial cysts than are the other regions.

3. Thoracic facet joints do not carry as much weight and are not subject to extensive torsional forces—hence they are less likely to develop osteoarthritis or synovial cysts.

4. Cervical facets do not carry much weight but are subject to extensive torsion. They are also quite prone to osteoarthritis but do not usually tend to form synovial cysts.

5. Synovial cysts, wherever they develop, are very well innervated with pain-conducting C fibers. They can be a source of arthritic pain. A

trial of lidocaine or steroid may afford temporary relief but is rarely curative.

6. If a synovial cyst were to cause symptoms of spinal stenosis, a trial of aspiration to decompress may be helpful. Decompressive surgery is indicated.

7. Synovial cyst walls commonly calcify, a fact much more readily apparent on CT than on MR imaging. Calcified cysts will be difficult to enter with a needle and probably cannot be decompressed percutaneously.

8. A synovial cyst that more superficially arises from the dorsolateral margin of a facet joint will present into the paraspinal musculature and not into the spinal canal and is much easier to approach and inject or drain.

V.   Equipment Requirements

A. Percutaneous drainage of a Tarlov, intraspinal arachnoid, or synovial cyst is typically performed under CT guidance, due to excellent depiction of the cyst and the adjacent osseous structures. The technique is similar to any CT-guided biopsy.

1. All of the aforementioned cysts are difficult to visualize under fluoroscopy, but fluoroscopic guidance could be used to locate the section of eroded sacrum that contains a Tarlov cyst. Intrathecal contrast injection may be helpful for visualizing all but the synovial cysts. Synovial cysts may show up well on fluoroscopy if they are calcified.

2. Overlying a Tarlov cyst there may be thinned but intact bone that cannot be visualized under fluoroscopy.

3. With the advent of MR-compatible needles and short sequences, MR-guided needle biopsies or aspirations are becoming possible.

4. While MR-guided aspiration of nerve root, Tarlov, arachnoid, and synovial cysts is possible, the advantages are not readily evident, and CT should be considered the modality of choice.

B. A 22 gauge 3.5 inch spinal needle is most useful for all of these interventions, although 18 and 20 gauge spinal needles can also be employed. Spinal needles are probably the best choice, as they are designed for puncturing the dura and entering the CSF space with a minimal amount of trauma.

1. 1% lidocaine without epinephrine is commonly all that is necessary as a local anesthetic, and a 3–5 ml Luer-Lok syringe can be helpful during aspiration maneuvers.

2. Betadine is used to clean the puncture site, and sterile towels drape the area in the usual manner.

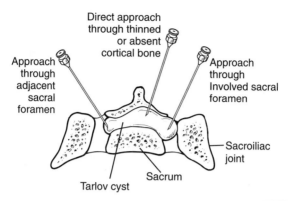

Figure 5–1. CT-guided drainage of Tarlov cyst. Demonstrates three possible approaches, depending on location of largest component of cyst(s).

3. Using CT-guidance, the spinal needle is directed to the outer edge of the target cyst and, after assuring location, pushed gently through the dura (Fig. 5–1). A characteristic myelographic "pop" can be felt.

4. If there is a thin lamella of bone overlying a Tarlov cyst, more force or a larger needle may be necessary to actually puncture the sacrum.

5. For nerve root cysts, needle placement is ideal at the point of largest diameter of the cyst, as determined on CT images obtained for localization (Fig. 5–2). The nerve root sheath may not be very thick at this location, and a "pop" may not be felt upon entering the cyst.

6. For a synovial cyst that is presenting into the spinal canal, or for an intraspinal arachoid cyst completely within the spinal canal, one must search several contiguous CT slices at the time of the procedure in order to find the best spot to enter the canal and avoid neural structures (Fig. 5–3).

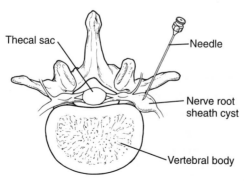

Figure 5–2. CT-guided drainage of peripheral nerve root sheath cyst: The lateral approach is usually sufficient. External nerve root is not a concern; such transient entry is harmless.

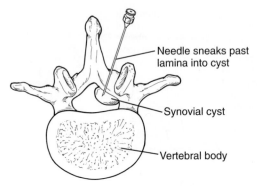

Figure 5–3. CT-guided synovial cyst drainage. Entering the cyst is often very difficult because of the location of cyst in relationship to lamina. A further complication might be calcification of cyst wall.

a. The patient may have to be placed with a pillow under the stomach to open up the posterior elements and accomplish this goal.

b. The needle placement is then again treated exactly like a CT-guided biopsy in any other crucial area of the body, with needle tip guidance afforded by triangulation and frequently obtained CT images along the way.

c. Cysts that communicate with the facet joint can be treated by performing a facet injection and do not need to be directly punctured.

VI.   Sedation

A. No sedation is typically necessary.

B. Patients may desire a mild relaxant such as Valium 5–10 mg p.o. or a tranquilizer of their own choice and from their own medicine cabinet, if high anxiety is present.

VII.   Procedure

A. For drainage of any of the cysts discussed, the patient is placed on the CT table in the prone position.

1. A bolster placed under the abdomen may be used to flatten the lumbosacral lordosis, making the neural foramina more perpendicular to the CT slice plane. Dorsal access to any of these cystic lesions is preferred.

2. A site is chosen after examination of preparatory scout CT scans. The

chosen level that allows direct access through the desired anatomical feature and the overlying skin is sterilized with Betadine.

3. If no direct access is present in the sacrum for a Tarlov cyst, it may be necessary to create a small hole with the needle through the thinnest part of the overlying bone. This access is typically easy to accomplish, as the overlying bone will almost always be paper thin or absent altogether.

4. 1% lidocaine is used for local anesthesia down to the periosteum or to the outer soft tissue layers of the spine. The needle is directed through into the cyst.

5. As with all spinal punctures there may be a slight amount of resistance when the outer surface of the cyst is encountered. The needle then is advanced a few millimeters into the cyst with a short, sharp push.

B. Following confirmation of appropriate needle placement in the cyst by a quick CT scan, the stylet is removed, and CSF is allowed to drain under its own pressure through the needle.

1. An extension tubing, with the proximal end lower than the needle hub, will speed the process. Patient improvement does not require removal of large amounts of CSF.

2. Gentle aspiration can be performed at the end of the drainage, although if the walls contact the needle tip in a CSF-filled cyst, the patient will have a sudden, sharp radiating pain. The exact radiation will depend on the location of the cyst.

   a. Warning the patient of this pain ahead of time will prevent deterioration of the patient-physician relationship. The pain typically should ease once the aspiration is ceased.

   b. The puncture site is cleaned and dressed with an adhesive bandage.

   c. The drainage procedure is terminated when CSF stops draining out of its own accord or when gentle aspiration creates patient pain.

C. Steroid injection into a nerve root sheath cyst or Tarlov cyst may theoretically encourage sclerosis of the cyst but is not recommended or universally accepted at the time of this writing, due to the risk of arachnoiditis from accidental intrathecal leakage.

D. Fibrin glue injection is not recommended on nerve root or Tarlov cysts due to the risk of aseptic meningitis.

E. For synovial cyst needle placement, the patient is placed on the table and the skin prepped in exactly the same manner as described above.

F. If the synovial cyst is in the cervical or thoracic areas, it is best to avoid draining it. These are surgical lesions.

G. If the synovial cyst is in the lumbar area, as the greatest majority of them are, then proceed as follows:

1. Find, using contiguous CT slices, a level that allows access to the cyst without the lamina being in the way. Many of these cysts freely communicate with the facet joint and can be drained by placing a needle into the joint, rather than the cyst.

2. Intrathecal contrast may be necessary to visualize the cyst in relationship to the rest of the thecal sac and its contents.

3. If the cyst is calcified, it will be easy to visualize but difficult to puncture.

4. Entering the cyst dorsally will result in a palpable "pop" as the wall of the cyst is punctured.

5. Synovial fluid may be viscous and will probably require aspiration.

6. A small amount (0.1–0.3 ml) of intracystic steroid deposition (Celestone or equivalent) may help to calm the inflammatory process that is the origin of these cysts.

7. Intrafacet steroid injection can be beneficial in those cysts that communicate with the joint space, resulting in cyst resolution in approximately one third of cases.[16]

H. If the synovial cyst presents dorsolaterally to the facet joint, outside of the spinal canal, the approach and subsequent puncture are much easier. It should be approached like a facet block (see Chapter 4).

I. The number of images obtained is at the discretion of the operator for any of the cyst punctures just described, but only a localizer tomogram and the final picture, with the needle in the cyst, may be necessary.

1. The main objective for taking a CT slice or fluoroscopic spot film is to create a permanent record to avoid future question as to the exact location of the tip of the needle at the time of drainage.

2. These images are to be considered mandatory. If the operator does not make a permanent record of the procedure, there is no proof that it happened exactly the way he/she knows that it did.

VIII.   Post-procedure Care

A. Patients can leave immediately following any of these puncture procedures, with reduced activities or bedrest at home encouraged for 6–12 hours.

B. Although CSF leak has not been reported from percutaneous drainage of any of the nerve root sheath cysts or Tarlov cyst, it is a theoretical possibility.

C. The patient is instructed to report any increasing back pain, fever, headache, nausea, or vomiting. A telephone number to reach the physician after hours is provided.

IX.   Procedure Reporting

A. The report should include a rationale for the procedure in the particular patient under consideration, emphasizing that the diagnostic information obtained could determine if the patient is a surgical candidate.

B. A complete description of the consent process and the procedure should follow, including worst-case scenarios. No reported fatalities from any of these procedures are currently known. A quantitative description of the volume of aspirated CSF should be included.

C. In patients who present with radiculopathy or more diffuse types of pain, an immediate objective assessment can be made regarding symptomatic relief immediately following the procedure and should be included in the report.

D. In patients with incontinence, an immediate determination of the efficacy of the procedure may not be possible while the patient is at the hospital, and follow-up phone calls to the patient perhaps as soon as 24 hours afterward should be made and documented.

E. As some clinicians at the time of this writing may be unfamiliar with Tarlov or nerve root cyst aspiration procedures, a sentence regarding the temporary nature of symptomatic relief following the procedure should be included.

X.   Coding

A. Although there is not a specific CPT code for spinal nerve root cyst aspiration, Tarlov cyst aspiration, or intraspinal arachnoid cyst aspiration, the most appropriate 2001 CPT codes would be 62272 (Spinal puncture, therapeutic, for drainage of spinal fluid) and 76360 (Computerized tomography guidance for needle placement).

B. If fluoroscopic or MR guidance were used, the latter code would be replaced with the guidance code for the appropriate imaging modality.

C. Synovial cyst drainage and steroid injection should be coded as 64475 (Lumbar Facet) whether the cyst was drained by direct puncture or through the facet, as the cysts originate from the joint space. Again, the appropriate guidance code should be used.

SUGGESTED READING

1. Tarlov IM: Perineural cysts of the spine nerve roots. Arch Neurol Psychiatry 40:1067–1074, 1938.

2. Paulsen RD, Call GA, Murtagh FR: Prevalence and percutaneous drainage of cysts of the sacral nerve root sleeve (Tarlov cysts). AJNR 15:293–297, 1994.
3. Naidich TP, McLone DG, Harwood-Nash DC: Arachnoid cysts, paravertebral meningoceles and perineural cysts. In Newton TH, Potts DG (eds): Modern Neuroradiology, vol 1. Computed Tomography of the Spine and Spinal Cord. San Anselmo, CA, Clavadel Press, 1983, pp 383–396.
4. Hodges SC: Arachnoid (meningeal) cysts. In St. Amour TE, Hodges SC, Laakman RW (eds): MRI of the Spine. New York, Raven Press, 1994.
5. Shreiber F, Haddad B: Lumbar and sacral cysts causing pain. J Neurosurg 8:504–509, 1951.
6. Tarlov IM: Sacral nerve-root cysts. Another cause of the sciatic or cauda-equina syndrome. Springfield, Charles C Thomas, 1953.
7. Wilkins RH: Commentary on prevalence and percutaneous drainage of cysts of the sacral nerve root sleeve (Tarlov cysts). AJNR 15:298–299, 1994.
8. Patel MR, Louie W, Rachlin J: Percutaneous fibrin glue therapy of meningeal cysts of the sacral spine. AJR Am J Roentgenol 168:367–370, 1997.
9. Bartels RH, van Overbeeke JJ: Lumbar cerebrospinal fluid drainage for symptomatic sacral nerve root cysts: an adjuvant diagnostic procedure and/or alternative treatment? Technical case report. Neurosurgery 40:861–864, 1997.
10. Mummaneni PV, Pitts LH, McCormack BM, et al: Microsurgical treatment of symptomatic Tarlov cysts. Neurosurgery 47:74–78, 2000.
11. Nabors MW, Pait TG, Byrd EB, et al: Updated assessment and current classification of spinal meningeal cysts. J Neurosurg 68:366–377, 1988.
12. Tarlov IM: Cysts (perineurial) of the sacral nerve roots: Another cause (removable) of sciatic pain. JAMA 138:740–744, 1948.
13. Fortuna A, La Torre E, Ciappetta P: Arachnoid diverticula: a unitary approach to spinal cysts communicating with the subarachnoid space. Acta Neurochir 39:259–268, 1977.
14. Tsuchiya K, Katase S, Hachiya J: MR myelography of sacral meningeal cysts. Acta Radiologica 40:95–99, 1999.
15. Boukobza M, Sichez JP, Rolland E, et al: MRI evaluation of sacral cysts. J Neuroradiol 20:266–271, 1993.
16. Parlier-Cuau C, Wybier M, Nizard R, et al: Symptomatic lumbar facet joint synovial cysts: Clinical assessment of facet joint steroid injection after 1 and 6 months and long-term follow-up in 30 patients. Radiology 210:509–513, 1999.

Other Recommended Reading

Wilkins RH, Odom GL: Spinal extradural cysts. In Inken PJ, Bruyn GW (eds): Handbook of Clinical Neurology, vol. 20. Tumors of the Spine and Spinal Cord. Part II. Amsterdam, North-Holland, 1976, pp 137–175.

6

Myelography

Alan L. Williams, M.D.

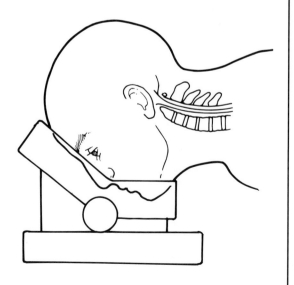

I. Rationale for Procedure and Clinical Indications

A. Myelography in one form or another has been around since 1921. The advent of magnetic resonance (MR) imaging of the spine has lessened, but not eliminated, the need for myelography. For one reason or another some patients are not candidates for MR (or MR is not available); thus the radiologist must be able to perform a myelogram safely and efficiently so that a diagnostic procedure can result.

B. Clinical indications for myelography include but are not limited to:

1. Use of MR being contraindicated (the presence of a pacemaker, neurostimulator, certain aneurysm clips, obesity, or claustrophobia)

2. Presence of surgical hardware in the area of interest producing artifacts on MR that preclude a diagnostic examination

3. Need for evaluation of an equivocal MR finding

4. Assessment of lumbar instability and stenosis utilizing dynamic (flexion and/or extension) techniques

II. Contraindications to Myelography

A. Some contraindications are relative while others are virtually absolute. It is the responsibility of the radiologist and the referring physician to weigh the risks and benefits of myelography and the availability of other, less potentially harmful studies to obtain the needed diagnostic information.

B. Contraindications include but are not limited to:

1. Allergy to iodinated contrast agents

2. Seizure disorder

3. Medications that lower the seizure threshold
   a. Phenothiazine derivatives (e.g., Compazine, Stelazine, Thorazine)
   b. Tricyclic antidepressants (e.g., Elavil, Sinequan)
   c. Monoamine oxidase (MAO) inhibitors (e.g., Nardil, Parnate)
   d. CNS stimulants
   e. Analeptics
   f. Antipsychotic agents

4. Blood modifier medications
   a. anticoagulants (e.g., Coumadin, heparin)
   b. antiplatelet agents (e.g., ReoPro)

5. Elevated intracranial pressure (e.g., brain tumor); potential risk of tonsillar herniation with lumbar puncture

6. Uncooperative patient

7. Pregnancy

III.   Informed Consent

A. Because a myelogram is not completely risk-free, informed consent must be obtained from the patient prior to proceeding with the myelogram.

B. The most common complication of myelography is post–lumbar puncture headache. The use of smaller-gauge needles, especially in an outpatient setting, has served to reduce the incidence of post-myelogram headaches.

C. Seizures related to contrast agents have become less frequent in the past 10–15 years as the agents have become less neurotoxic. However, patients must be informed that a seizure may result during or after myelography.

D. Other potential side effects of myelography include nausea, vomiting, musculoskeletal pain, allergy to the contrast agent, bleeding at the puncture site, infection, arachnoiditis, and nerve root injury.

E. When the lateral C1–2 approach is used, injury to the spinal cord is possible, and this rare complication should be discussed with the patient. This is an opportunity for the radiologist to impress upon the patient the need for complete cooperation during the course of the examination.

IV.   Pertinent Anatomy

A. Lumbar approach

1. A generous vertebral canal and thecal sac facilitate a successful puncture, and the likelihood of striking a nerve root with the needle tip is reduced.

2. The L2–3 level is generally preferred because there is less likelihood of a protruding disc and/or a stenotic canal at this level than at the L5–S1, L4–5, and L3–4 levels.

3. For a midline approach, the needle is passed through the supraspinous and interspinous ligaments, through the junction of the ligamenta flava into the posterior epidural space, and through the dura and arachnoid membrane into the subarachnoid space (Fig. 6–1).

4. The needle should be passed gently through the dura. If a nerve root is encountered with the needle tip, a brief "nudge" is preferable to an aggressive "thrust" from the patient's standpoint.

B. Lateral C1–2 approach

1. The posterior subarachnoid space at the C1–2 level tends to be

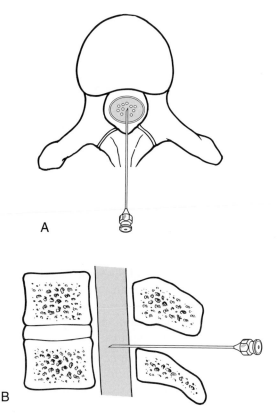

Figure 6–1. Normal anatomy pertinent to lumbar puncture in axial (*A*) and sagittal (*B*) planes.

generous in most patients, thus providing an adequate target for the needle (Fig. 6–2).

2. The spinal cord occupies approximately 50% of the subarachnoid space at the C1–2 level; thus the spectre of penetrating the cord with the needle is always present.

3. Needless to say, an expanded spinal cord or low-lying cerebellar tonsils could compromise an otherwise successful lateral C1–2 puncture. If available, a previous MR or CT scan demonstrating the craniocervical junction can be extremely helpful to the operator who is contemplating a lateral C1–2 puncture. MR may also identify a posterior inferior cerebellar artery (PICA) loop that can sometimes reach the C1–2 level.

V.   Equipment

A. Fluoroscopy unit

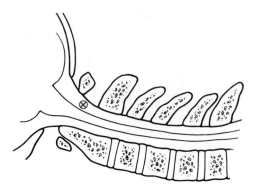

Figure 6–2. Normal anatomy pertinent to lateral C1–2 puncture in the sagittal plane. The needle target ⊗ is the junction of the middle and posterior one-third of the vertebral canal in order to avoid striking the spinal cord.

1. The standard Radiographic and Fluoroscopic (R and F) unit has been a staple of myelography for many years. The table must have 30-degree to 90-degree capability, that is minimum head-down tilt of at least 30 degrees and 90 degrees upright capability so that the patient can stand as the procedure requires.

2. The fluoroscopic unit must have small focal spot capability (0.6–1.0 mm), with collimation that should be both automatic and manual. The fluoroscopy tube should be rated at 70 kW or above for satisfactory motion-stopping imaging. The R and F unit's generator should have operating power of 80 kW (1000 mA maximum). Digital fluoroscopy is making its way into the myelography suite and limits the need for bulky cassettes that require exchanges during the crucial portions of the procedure.

B. Ankle restraints, boots, or shoulder bars are required for cervical myelography to prevent the patient from sliding when the table is tilted head-down to maneuver the contrast agent into the cervical subarachnoid space.

C. Cross-table lateral radiographic capability is facilitated with a cassette holder that maintains the cassette in a vertical position. A grid is required with the cassette to minimize scatter. Typical multipurpose grids have 8:1 ratio, 34–44″ focal range, and 85 lines per inch.

D. The lead apron that attaches to the fluoroscopy unit to minimize scatter to the operator should be in place when he or she is performing lumbar puncture and obtaining spot films. This apron may interfere with the operator attempting a lateral C1–2 puncture and should be removed prior to beginning the cervical puncture.

E. Head holder: For cervical myelograms, once the contrast has been instilled in the subarachnoid space, a head holder (e.g., Osborne head

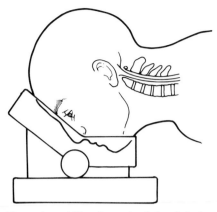

Figure 6–3. Head holder to immobilize the patient's head during cervical myelography.

support—Model 100, MG Medical Equipment Co., Inc., St. Paul, MN) maintains the prone patient in a comfortable hyperextended position during the imaging portion of the examination (Fig. 6–3). Alternatively, a cooperative patient may be positioned with the chin hyperextended on a sponge, sandbag, or towel roll (although there is a greater chance for the patient to move when not restrained by a head holder).

F. Rectangular sponge: Placed under the patient's head when he or she is positioned in lateral decubitus position for a C1–2 puncture using vertical fluoroscopy to position the needle.

G. Needles: There has been a trend over the past 8–10 years to use smaller-gauge spinal needles. A 3½ inch spinal needle is standard length. However, 20–22 gauge needles have given way to 24–26 gauge needles, especially in outpatient settings, for lumbar punctures to minimize post-myelogram headaches. Some operators use an 18-gauge needle in the subcutaneous tissues as a guide through which to pass the smaller spinal needle (Fig. 6–4).

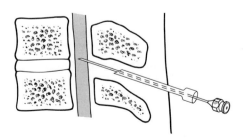

Figure 6–4. Coaxial technique facilitating utilization of small-gauge spinal needle for lumbar puncture.

H. Myelography tray: May be purchased or put together piecemeal. The tray should include:

1. Swabs (3) for "painting" the antiseptic solution on the skin
2. Gauze sponges (4 × 4's).
3. Fenestrated drape
4. Paper towel for removing excess antiseptic solution
5. Syringes:
   a. 5 ml—for local anesthetic
   b. 20 ml—for contrast agent
6. Clear flexible 50 cm plastic tubing
7. Test tubes (3) with tight-sealing caps when cerebrospinal fluid (CSF) studies are desired.

I. Surgical gloves:

1. Powder should be wiped from the gloves using alcohol or sterile saline.
   a. Experimental studies in dogs have demonstrated the presence of powder from surgical gloves in the subarachnoid space following myelography via lumbar puncture.
   b. Thus, glove powder is a potential source of adhesive arachnoiditis.

J. Contrast agents

1. Virtually all myelography now utilizes water-soluble nonionic agents that possess substantially less neurotoxicity than the earlier water-soluble agents.
2. Common nonionic water-soluble contrast agents in clinical use today: iopamidol (Isovue) and iohexol (Omnipaque).
3. Conventional contrast agent concentrations:
   a. Lumbar and thoracic: 180–240 mgI/ml
   b. Cervical myelogram: 240–300 mgI/ml
4. Iophendylate (Pantopaque), a myelographic staple for decades, is no longer on the market. This oil-based agent was not water-soluble and had to be aspirated by the operator at the conclusion of the myelogram. Given the availability of MR imagers and water-soluble contrast agents, it is difficult to conceive of an indication for Pantopaque myelography today.

VI. Sedation

A. For most patients undergoing myelography, sedation is *not* required. Discussing the procedure in a calm, reassuring manner and providing an opportunity to answer the patient's questions usually helps alleviate the patient's anxiety and obviates the need for sedation. Atropine sulfate, an anticholinergic, is used by some operators to reduce the likelihood of a vasovagal reaction. Dosage: 0.4–1.0 mg IV. Contraindications to atropine include glaucoma and heart disease.

B. For the extremely anxious patient, *conscious sedation* may be appropriate.

1. Conscious sedation should be conducted in accordance with each facility's conscious sedation policy.

2. Benzodiazepines commonly used include:

    a. Midazolam (Versed)—has anxiolytic and amnestic properties. Dosage: 0.5–3.0 mg IV. Beware the potential for respiratory depression, especially in the elderly.

    b. Diazepam (Valium)—an anxiolytic. Dosage: 2–10 mg IV. Do not use small veins such as those on the dorsum of the hand. Replaced by midazolam in many facilities.

3. Monitoring with continuous pulse oximetry is mandatory when conscious sedation is used. Parameters to be monitored and recorded include level of consciousness, respiratory rate, heart rate, blood pressure, and oxygen saturation. These parameters should be documented in the patient's medical record.

4. Supervisory personnel (physicians, nurses, technologists) should be certified in basic cardiac life support (BCLS) and, preferably, advanced cardiac life support (ACLS).

5. Drugs such as flumazenil (Romazicon), a benzodiazepine-receptor antagonist, should be readily available to reverse the sedation should the need arise.

6. Patients undergoing conscious sedation must be monitored following the myelogram for a minimum of 30–60 minutes after the last dose. These patients should not operate a motor vehicle or other machinery for 24 hours.

C. Agitated and/or uncooperative patients are not suitable candidates for myelography. If myelography is necessary in these patients, a representative of the department of anesthesiology should be consulted regarding General Anesthesia or "Anesthesia Standby."

D. A commonly used protocol for patients undergoing myelography with a history of previous contrast reaction:

1. Prednisone 32–50 mg P.O. at 12 and 2 hours prior to the procedure

2. Benadryl 50 mg P.O. one hour prior to (or 25 mg intravenously just preceding) the procedure

VII. Procedures

A. The operator should review all available imaging studies involving the area of interest prior to commencing the myelogram. Important imaging studies include plain radiographs, CT scans, MR scans, and myelograms.

1. Stenotic levels, herniated discs, neoplasms, and hematomas should and can be avoided.

2. Select the puncture level to avoid areas of known or suspected pathology.

3. If the area of interest is lumbar but the pathologic process is diffuse (e.g, hematoma, arachnoiditis), consider a lateral C1–2 puncture.

4. If a lateral C1–2 puncture is planned, a CT or MR scan depicting the region will ensure that low-lying cerebellar tonsils are identified.

5. Before lumbar puncture is performed, be sure that the patient does not have an intracranial mass. Lumbar puncture with its potential for lowering the intrathecal pressure carries an increased risk of tonsillar herniation in patients with a large intracranial mass, especially if it is located in the posterior fossa.

B. Laboratory studies

1. *Prior* to the myelogram:

   a. Normally no laboratory studies are required.

   b. If there is a question regarding renal function, serum creatinine and BUN may be obtained.

   c. If the patient has been on anticoagulants, obtain a coagulation panel including PT (prothrombin time), PTT (partial thromboplastin time), platelets, and INR (international normalizing ratio).

2. CSF studies

   a. Small-gauge needles currently used for most myelography preclude the acquisition of CSF for laboratory studies.

   b. If CSF studies are desired, the operator should use a 20 or 22 gauge needle.

   c. CSF studies generally require 5–10 ml of fluid, occasionally more.

   d. Common CSF laboratory studies include cell count, total protein, glucose, Gram stain, and culture.

   e. The operator should note CSF color (colorless, xanthochromic, bloody) and clarity (clear, cloudy) and comment on same in the myelography report.

   f. The operator should ensure that CSF specimens are clearly labeled with the patient name and hospital number and transported promptly to the laboratory with the appropriate request form.

C. Patient positioning for lumbar puncture

1. Prone; verify that the patient is not rotated. Use the fluoroscope to be sure that the spinous processes are centered between the pedicles.

2. Some operators use a towel roll under the abdomen to increase the interspinous distance and facilitate needle placement in the vertebral canal. However, this "abdominal compression" may restrict venous return from the pelvis and lower extremities and increase the likelihood of a vasovagal reaction, especially in thin patients.

3. For thoracic or cervical myelograms when the table will be tilted head-down, restraint "boots," ankle straps, or shoulder bars must be installed before the puncture begins.

D. Lateral C1–2 puncture

1. This technique is used routinely for cervical myelography by some radiologists.

2. It may also be used if direct access to the lumbar subarachnoid space is denied (e.g., infection, trauma, hematoma, stenosis) or if a "block" is present.

3. Positioning options

a. *Prone* with the cervical spine hyperextended on a sponge or towel roll (active hyperextension only by the patient; in a patient with cervical stenosis and spondylosis, passive hyperextension has resulted in spinal cord injury).

(1) In older patients, hyperextension must be conducted with great care.

(2) Needle localization and puncture may be conducted with cross-table (horizontal beam) fluoroscopy or using a portable radiography machine, which can be time-consuming (see Fig. 6–2).

b. *Right lateral (right side down) decubitus* (which permits needle to be on same side of patient as the radiologist when the patient is turned to prone position prior to injecting contrast agent).

(1) Cervical spine in neutral position

(2) Head resting on a sponge or towel roll with the cervical spine parallel to the tabletop and the angles of the mandible superimposed (Fig. 6–5)

E. *Lumbar myelogram* utilizing lumbar puncture

1. Palpate the interspinous space at desired level. L2–3 is the preferred level if there is no contraindication (e.g., herniated disc, intraspinal mass, superficial infection, and the like) because it is rostral to most herniated discs and stenoses.

2. Make an indentation in the skin with thumbnail between the spi-

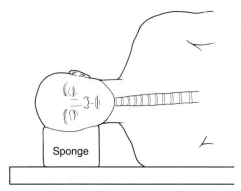

Figure 6–5. Lateral decubitus positioning of a patient for lateral C1–2 puncture utilizing vertical fluoroscopy.

nous processes at the desired level (or use a marker pen if the patient is large and fluoroscopy is used to localize the puncture site).

3. Skin preparation:

a. Shave hair as necessary for 25–30 cm hair-free area.

b. Use a topical antiseptic, bactericidal agent such as Betadine (povidone-iodine) solution to prepare the skin; let the Betadine remain on the skin surface while setting up myelogram equipment because the maximal antibacterial effect takes several minutes.

c. Blot off excess Betadine with a sterile towel.

d. Swab the prepared area with isopropyl alcohol and dry with sterile towel or sponge.

e. Be sure to wipe surgical gloves with alcohol or sterile saline to remove powder.

f. Place sterile fenestrated drape over the puncture site. Ensure that the drape access provides for a potential puncture at two or three levels in case of a problem at the initial puncture site.

4. Sterility of the fluoroscopic unit: Ensure that a sterile drape or towel covers the fluoroscopy unit handle and controls so that the operator may maneuver the fluoroscope while maintaining sterility.

5. Local anesthesia

a. With 1-cm 25-gauge needle, infiltrate the skin at the marked location. Use 2.5-cm 25-gauge needle to infiltrate deeper tissues.

b. With the advent of 25-gauge and 26-gauge spinal needles, some operators no longer anesthetize the skin and subcutaneous tissues, rationalizing that raising a wheal and infiltrating the superficial soft tissues with the local anesthetic is more painful than using the small-gauge spinal needle without anesthetic.

   c. Xylocaine 1% or a similar agent is commonly used.

   d. 3–5 ml of anesthetic agent is usually sufficient to anesthetize the superficial soft tissues.

6. Spinal needle placement for lumbar puncture

   a. *Midline approach*

     (1) Start the needle in the midline at the anesthetized level and use frequent, short (1–3 sec) checks with the fluoroscope to monitor needle position.

     (2) Be careful not to strike the needle with the fluoroscope tower (set tower lock to ensure needle clearance prior to commencing puncture).

     (3) At L2–3 level the needle path will be essentially vertical; at the L3–4 level, some cephalad direction will be required.

     (4) Needles smaller than 20 gauge will usually not produce a "pop" (abrupt "give" felt by the operator) when passing through the dura. The needle tip depth may be checked with a cross-table lateral radiograph or cross-table fluoroscopy if the operator has a question as to needle location.

   b. *Oblique approach*

     (1) With the patient prone or slightly obliqued, start the needle at the inner margin of the pedicle.

     (2) Angle it medially and inferiorly between the laminae into the thecal sac.

7. Needle placement for lateral C1–2 puncture

   a. C-arm or cross-table fluoroscopy facilitates the puncture with the patient in prone position.

   b. Use 25 gauge 1 cm anesthetic needle as marker.

   c. The "target" is the junction of the middle and posterior one-third of the vertebral canal at the C1–2 level (see Fig. 6–2); this needle position should avoid the spinal cord and ensure entry into the posterior subarachnoid space.

8. Removal of CSF for laboratory studies

   a. Attach flexible 50-cm plastic tubing to the needle hub.

   b. When a 20–22 gauge needle is used for lumbar puncture, CSF usually flows spontaneously when the needle tip is in the subarachnoid space, especially if the table head is elevated 10–15 degrees.

   c. If CSF flow is poor, elevate the head of the table to 30–40 degrees.

d. If flow is still poor, gently rotate the needle hub 90–180 degrees.

e. The amount of CSF to be removed will depend on the laboratory studies desired. For "standard" studies (cell count, chemistry, and culture), 3–5 ml is usually sufficient.

f. When smaller spinal needles (24–27 gauge) are used, CSF aspiration is virtually impossible and is generally not performed.

g. Currently for most myelograms, CSF is no longer obtained for laboratory studies.

9. Instillation of contrast material via lumbar puncture

a. Once the needle tip is positioned within the subarachnoid space, remove the stylet and attach the flexible tubing connected to the syringe containing the contrast material to the needle hub. Inject a small amount (0.5–1.0 ml) of contrast while observing the needle under fluoroscopy. A subdural injection must be recognized promptly and the needle repositioned at another interspace if the examination is to be technically satisfactory.

b. Be sure that the contrast agent is seen filling the dependent nerve root sheaths, and cauda equina nerve roots can be visualized surrounded by contrast agent before injecting entire contrast volume. When injecting the contrast agent, check intermittently with the fluoroscope to ensure that the agent continues to flow only into the subarachnoid space.

c. The contrast volume utilized will depend on the size of the thecal sac and the regions of the spine to be studied. Use the minimum amount of contrast agent necessary to opacify the subarachnoid space in the region of interest. Typical contrast agent concentrations and volumes are as follows:

(1) Lumbar myelogram: 180–240 mgI/ml; 10–15 ml

(2) Thoracic myelogram: 180–240 mgI/ml; 10–15 ml

(3) Cervical myelogram: 240–300 mgI/ml; 10 ml

d. Some operators take an AP spot film of the lumbar spine prior to removing the needle to assist in recognition of any iatrogenic extradural defect associated with the needle.

e. Prior to the imaging portion of the myelogram, remove the needle carefully; remove the drapes and place a Band-Aid over the puncture site. Reassure the patient that the remainder of the study is painless and remind him or her that it is important to follow your instructions regarding positioning and breathing to the best of his or her ability.

10. Imaging portion of the lumbar myelogram: with the head of the table elevated 30–40 degrees, the operator should obtain the following spot films:

a. One-on-one AP spot film without collimation to include the sacrum and iliac crest. This film proves useful when documenting a transitional vertebra at the lumbosacral junction and determining the proper numbering of each vertebra (e.g., L4, L5, S1, and so on).

b. AP spot film(s) with tight collimation to the contrast column to minimize scattered radiation

c. Two-on-one graded (30–60 degree) oblique (RPO and LPO) spot films with relatively tight collimation to the contrast column

d. Lateral spot films with the table head elevated to 90 degrees with the patient in neutral, flexion, and extension

e. Cross-table lateral radiograph by the technologist:

   (1) The technologist should have obtained a preliminary scout film to ensure optimal technique prior to beginning the myelogram.

   (2) Table head elevation is generally limited to 10–20 degrees.

   (3) Swimmer's view is frequently necessary to image the cervicothoracic junction adequately in large patients.

11. Imaging the conus medullaris:

    a. When the lumbar subarachnoid space has been examined satisfactorily (images approved by the operating radiologist), the patient may be turned to the lateral decubitus position (or maintained in the prone position).

    b. The head of the table is then tilted down 10–15 degrees, and contrast within the lumbar subarachnoid space observed under fluoroscopy.

    c. The contrast will move cephalad more quickly with the patient in the decubitus position, since the spine is now parallel to the tabletop (except in patients with scoliosis).

    d. When the conus can be seen outlined by the contrast material, raise the head of the table enough to stabilize the contrast column, then obtain collimated (side to side) spot films of the thoracolumbar junction.

    e. If imaging of the entire thoracic subarachnoid space is not desired, the table head may be quickly brought back to the horizontal position or elevated to 10–20 degrees to prevent the contrast from cascading into the thoracic, cervical, or even the intracranial subarachnoid space.

12. Once imaging is completed, the contrast material should be collected in the lumbosacral region and the patient maintained in a

30-degree head-elevated position before being sent for the usual post-myelogram CT scan.

F. *Lumbar myelogram* utilizing the *lateral C1–2 approach*

1. Place the patient prone in either right- or left-side down lateral decubitus position as noted under the Procedures section. The lateral decubitus position permits the use of the vertical fluoroscopic capability of an R and F unit.

2. A 22-gauge spinal needle is a nice compromise of caliber and directability.

3. Once a successful puncture is achieved, maintain the patient in the lateral decubitus position and connect flexible tubing to the needle hub.

4. Raise the head of the table 20–30 degrees.

5. If CSF is required for laboratory analysis, it should be obtained at this time.

6. Then connect the syringe with the contrast agent to the tubing and slowly inject 2–3 ml under fluoroscopic visualization, ensuring that the contrast is subarachnoid and streaming caudal in the dependent lateral subarachnoid space.

   a. Use the fluoroscope to ensure that the contrast agent is collecting in the lumbosacral region rather than being obstructed in the cervical, thoracic, or upper lumbar region.

   b. Generally 15–17 ml of contrast agent (180–240 mgI/ml concentration) is preferable with this approach because some of the contrast agent will diffuse into the CSF in the cervical and thoracic subarachnoid spaces.

7. Once the entire volume of contrast has been instilled, remove the needle, turn the patient into the prone position, and proceed with the imaging as per the lumbar approach.

G. *Thoracic Myelogram*

1. Although the needle puncture and instillation of contrast agent is typically via the lumbar approach, the lateral C1–2 approach may be used if the lumbar puncture is unsuccessful or contraindicated.

2. If the lumbar approach is employed, once the contrast is within the lumbosacral subarachnoid space, the patient is turned from the prone to the *lateral decubitus position*.

3. Ensuring that the patient's feet, ankles, or shoulders are anchored so that he or she will not slide on the table, tilt the head of the table down 10–20 degrees, frequently observing the contrast column via fluoroscopy.

4. When the bulk of the contrast has entered the thoracic subarachnoid

space, quickly return the table to the horizontal position and turn the patient supine, thus "capturing" the contrast in the dependent kyphotic curve of the thoracic spine.

5. Be attentive to the contrast column at all times because the agent can quickly pass through the thoracic subarachnoid space into the cervical subarachnoid space and even into the intracranial subarachnoid space.

6. With the patient in the lateral decubitus position, his or her head should be elevated on sponges to produce lateral cervical spine tilt so that any contrast escaping the thoracic subarachnoid space will be trapped in the cervical region rather than egressing into the intracranial compartment.

7. *Thoracic myelogram* via lateral C1–2 puncture

   a. Options include the *prone* position utilizing cross-table fluoroscopy or radiography, or the *lateral decubitus* position using vertical fluoroscopy.

   b. If the lateral decubitus position is selected, consider left-side down in case the operator wants to rotate the patient into the supine position before completing the instillation of contrast.

   c. Instill the contrast slowly under fluoroscopic visualization to ensure that the contrast is in the subarachnoid space.

   d. If the patient is in lateral decubitus position, it will not require much table head-up (10–15 degrees) to move the contrast into the thoracic subarachnoid space. However, the tendency will be for the contrast to keep moving caudad from the thoracic into the lumbar subarachnoid space.

   e. Turn the patient supine to capture the contrast in the kyphotic curvature of the thoracic spine.

   f. If the contrast moves too quickly and it ends up in the lumbar region, stand the patient up to collect all the contrast in the lumbosacral region. Then place the patient decubitus and tilt the table head-down 10–15 degrees and observe under fluoroscopy the contrast column moving into the thoracic subarachnoid space.

8. Imaging portion of the thoracic myelogram

   a. AP and cross-table lateral radiographs provide excellent definition of the thoracic subarachnoid space and spinal cord.

   b. AP or oblique spot films may be obtained as necessary.

H. *Cervical Myelogram*

   1. Either the lumbar or lateral C1–2 route is appropriate.

   2. The lateral C1–2 approach has the advantage of instilling the contrast agent directly into the area of interest in high concentration

and maintaining the table in the horizontal position (or nearly so), thus minimizing the likelihood of spilling contrast material into the intracranial subarachnoid space with the potential sequelae of headache, nausea, vomiting, and seizures.

3. In the lateral C1–2 approach, the patient is prone and the table horizontal.

4. As the contrast is injected, monitoring via fluoroscopy is mandatory, as a block in the mid or lower cervical region (e.g., central stenosis, disc herniation, tumor) must be recognized quickly; otherwise, there is a real risk of contrast backing up from the level of the block in the cervical region into the intracranial compartment.

5. If the lumbar route has been selected and contrast material is instilled into the lumbar subarachnoid space, the procedure for cervical myelography is similar to that for the thoracic. That is, the patient is turned into the lateral decubitus position and the patient's head is elevated with sponges to produce moderate lateral cervical spine tilt (Fig. 6–6).

6. The contrast is then maneuvered into the cervical subarachnoid space utilizing head-down table tilt (monitoring the contrast via fluoroscopy as it moves from the lumbar through the thoracic into the cervical subarachnoid space). *Be careful* not to strike the patient's head with the fluoroscope tower as you follow the contrast column!

7. Once the contrast is trapped in the cervical subarachnoid space, the patient's cervical spine is gently hyperextended; the patient is then rolled into the prone position and the head is placed in a head holder (or with the chin on a sponge or sandbag).

8. If the patient is maintained in the *prone* position rather than lateral

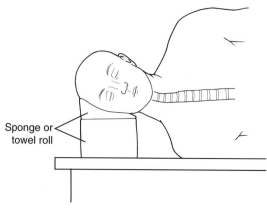

Sponge or
towel roll

Figure 6–6. Patient positioning to prevent spillage of contrast agent into the intracranial subarachnoid space when performing cervical myelography via lumbar puncture.

decubitus, the table will need to be tilted more head-down (15–30 degrees). Maintain the patient with the cervical spine hyperextended so the contrast agent will not enter the intracranial subarachnoid space. When the contrast has reached the cervical region, return the table to the horizontal position and place the patient in the head holder or maintain him or her in hyperextended position with chin on sponge or bolster.

9. Imaging portion of the cervical myelogram

 a. AP spot film to include the upper thoracic region for aid in numbering levels

 b. Oblique radiographs preferably utilizing an overhead x-ray tube, so the patient does not move from the prone hyperextended position (Fig. 6–7). Oblique images can also be obtained by having the patient turn slightly into the RPO and LPO positions;

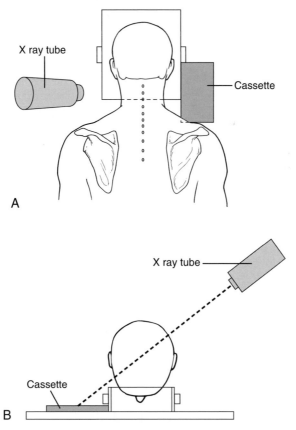

Figure 6–7. Cassette positioning for oblique filming during cervical myelogram. *A,* Viewed from above the patient. *B,* Viewed from in front of the patient.

however, the contrast agent has a tendency to migrate caudally or rostrally with patient movement.

    c. Cross-table lateral radiograph

    d. A lateral Swimmer's view is frequently used, especially in large patients, to image the cervicothoracic junction.

10. At the conclusion of the myelogram, the head of the table should be raised 45–60 degrees to allow the contrast to collect in the lumbosacral subarachnoid space. Sufficient contrast will remain in the cervical subarachnoid space to facilitate CT scanning immediately after myelography.

VIII. Post-procedure Care

A. Prior to post-myelogram CT scanning

1. The head of the gurney or bed should be elevated 30 degrees; alternatively, the patient may be seated in a chair.
2. The patient should be under observation by medical personnel (nurse, technologist, or physician) at all times.

B. Following post-myelogram CT scanning

1. The patient should be observed in the radiology department, ambulatory surgery unit, or some such facility for 1–4 hours after the myelogram.
2. Most operators prefer that their patients be sitting up or in bed with the head of the bed elevated at least 30 degrees for a minimum of six hours.

C. Prior to discharge

1. The patient should be instructed about activity, diet, oral fluids, and potential side effects such as headaches and seizures.
2. Patients should not be allowed to drive themselves home and should be accompanied at home by a competent adult for 24 hours after the myelogram.
3. When a large-gauge needle (20–22 gauge) is used, instructing the patient to lie flat after the initial six-hour "head up" period is designed to minimize the likelihood of the patient developing a post-myelogram headache.
4. The patient should be instructed to drink plenty of fluids over the next 24 hours.
5. The patient should be provided with the name and telephone number of the operating radiologist or a colleague having call responsibility in case a problem develops.

6. The patient should be instructed not to operate a motor vehicle or machinery for 24 hours.

D. Treating the "post-myelogram headache"

1. The "post-myelogram headache" is thought to be due to CSF leaking out of the lumbar puncture hole in the dural sac, lowering the pressure in the spinal subarachnoid space and causing settling of the brain within the cranial vault and meningeal stretching when the patient is in the erect position.

2. These headaches usually respond to having the patient lie flat in bed and drink plenty of fluids. Most CSF leaks seal spontaneously within 1–2 days following this supportive therapy.

3. If the headache persists for one week or more, performing a "blood patch" may be warranted.

   a. With the patient prone, insert a 22 gauge spinal needle into the posterior epidural space under fluoroscopic guidance at the level of the myelographic lumbar puncture, being careful not to advance the needle into the subarachnoid space.

   b. Perform an epidurogram by injecting a small amount (3–5 ml) of nonionic contrast under fluoroscopic guidance, thus ensuring that the needle is not subarachnoid and that the posterior epidural space is patent.

   c. Via venapuncture from one of the patient's antecubital veins, remove 10–15 ml of blood and inject it via flexible tubing connected to the needle hub into the posterior epidural space.

   d. Before injecting the autologous blood, be certain that you are not instilling blood into a stenotic vertebral canal, creating a mass that may seriously compromise the thecal sac and the cauda equina.

   e. The patient should be maintained in the horizontal position for four hours before being discharged home.

   f. The blood in the posterior epidural space usually seals the defect in the dura and relieves the patient's symptoms.

IX. Reporting the myelogram

A. The final myelogram report should include:

1. Patient name

2. Name of procedure (e.g., "cervical myelogram")

3. Date

4. Clinical history or indication for the study (e.g., low back pain, neck pain, left C6 radiculopathy, and the like)

5. Procedure technique

   a. Puncture site

   b. Name and amount of contrast agent

6. Findings

   a. Describe all intramedullary, intradural extramedullary and extra-dural abnormalities with specific detailing of levels involved.

   b. Mention any complication (e.g., vasovagal response, subdural injection, and so on).

7. Impression

   a. This should be a summary of key findings in descending order of clinical importance.

   b. Do not merely repeat the findings.

X. Myelogram coding

CPT Code

A. Procedural coding for puncture and injection of contrast agent

   1. Lateral cervical (C1–2)   61055

   2. Lumbar   62284

B. Myelogram supervision and interpretation

   1. Cervical   72240–26

   2. Thoracic   72255–26

   3. Lumbar   72265–26

   4. Complete (cervical, thoracic and lumbar)   72270–26

C. Post-myelogram CT scan supervision and interpretation

   1. Cervical   72126–26

   2. Thoracic   72129–26

   3. Lumbar   72132–26

SUGGESTED READING

1. Johansen JG, Orrison WW, Amundsen P: Lateral C1–2 puncture for cervical myelography. Part I: Report of a complication. Radiology 146:391–393, 1983.
2. Kovanen J, Sulkava R: Duration of postural headache after lumbar puncture: effect of needle size. Headache 26:224–226, 1986.
3. Newton TH, Potts DG: Modern Neuroradiology, Volume 1. Computed Tomography of the Spine and Spinal Cord. San Anselmo, CA, Clavadel Press, 1983.
4. Orrison WW, Sackett JF, Amundsen P: Lateral C1–2 puncture for cervical myelography. Part II: Recognition of improper injection of contrast material. Radiology 146:395–400, 1983.

5. Orrison WW, Eldevik OP, Sackett JF: Lateral C1–2 puncture for cervical myelography. Part III: Historical, anatomic and technical considerations. Radiology 146:401–408, 1983.
6. Peterman SB: Post-myelography headache: a review. Radiology 200:765–770, 1996.
7. Post MJD: Radiographic Evaluation of the Spine. New York, Masson Publishing USA, Inc., 1980.
8. Sackett JF, Strother CM: New techniques in myelography. Hagerstown, MD, Harper and Row, 1979.
9. Shapiro R: Myelography, 4th ed., Chicago, Year Book Medical Publishers, Inc., 1984.
10. Vezina JL, Fontaine S, Laperriere J: Out-patient myelography with fine-needle technique: an appraisal. AJR 153:383–385, 1989.

7

Percutaneous Needle Biopsy of the Spine

Glen K. Geremia, M.D.

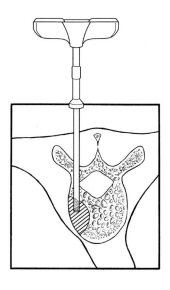

I. Clinical Indications for Vertebral Column Biopsy

A. Focal vertebral column lesion in a symptomatic or asymptomatic patient. Patients referred for biopsy often present with a chief complaint of back pain.

   1. The patient may have a lesion identified during a diagnostic workup that could include conventional radiology, computed tomography (CT), magnetic resonance imaging (MRI), or radionuclide bone scan.

   2. Some clinically silent lesions can be detected on a screening study in a patient with known primary tumor.

   3. Percutaneous CT-guided biopsy provides accurate specimen sampling in patients with a focal destructive lesion.

B. New vertebral body compression fracture in a patient with or without known tumor.

   1. This is especially noteworthy in elderly patients with a single vertebral body compression fracture and a known primary tumor that has been treated in the past.

   2. The dilemma is whether this represents a benign osteoporotic compression fracture or a pathologic fracture.

   3. Sometimes it is impossible to discern the malignant potential of a lesion based on radiographic or MRI studies alone.

C. Malignant-appearing lesion in a patient with known primary tumor to discern metastatic spread versus a new additional primary tumor.

D. Confirmation of clinically and radiographically suspected osteomyelitis or discitis. Patients with back pain who have radiographic findings consistent with osteomyelitis or discitis, for example, loss of intervertebral disc-space height, are also referred for biopsy.

E. Isolation of a pathologic organism in a patient with a diagnosis of osteomyelitis or discitis based on radiographic and clinical findings. The radiographic appearance may be consistent with infection; however, biopsy is necessary to isolate the offending organism.

II. Contraindications

A. Patient predisposed to hemorrhaging.

   1. A low platelet count, for example, $<50,000 \ mm^3$, increases the risk of bleeding from a biopsy.

   2. An abnormal coagulation profile with elevated prothrombin time and partial thromboplastin time.

   3. Transfusion with serum plasma and/or vitamin K may reverse these coagulopathies.

B. Uncooperative patient or one who cannot lie in the scanner for at least 20 minutes in order to properly position the spine biopsy needle.

III. Pre-procedure Workup and Informed Consent

This procedure is usually performed on an outpatient basis.

A. A brief medical history is taken, particularly emphasizing the patient's cardiac and respiratory status because intravenous sedation is administered. Any history of allergies to a medication or contrast agent is important.

B. The patient's current weight is necessary to determine the exact amount of intravenous sedation to administer.

C. Pre-procedural laboratory examinations
   1. Coagulation profile such as prothrombin time (PT), partial thromboplastin time (PTT), and a baseline complete blood count (CBC) with platelets. These baseline parameters are important because a hematoma at the biopsy site is a possible complication with this invasive procedure.
   2. Blood urea nitrogen (BUN) and creatinine levels are necessary if contrast medium is administered. Contrast is given to identify vascular structures when biopsying lesions within the cervical region.

D.
   1. Risks
      a. Infection
      b. Paralysis, partial or complete
      c. Acute and/or chronic localized and/or radicular pain
      d. Hematoma
      e. Reaction to administered drugs or contrast (when appropriate)
      f. Pneumothorax that may require placement of a chest tube when the thoracic spine is the biopsy site
   2. Expectations
      a. Mild discomfort due to position on CT table and duration of procedure (30–40 minutes)
      b. Minimal pain and moderate pressure sensation during needle advancement into bone.

IV. Sedation

A. Conscious monitored intravenous sedation provides pain and anxiety relief to the patient. Continuous monitored sedation can be attained with the intravenous use of fentanyl citrate or midazolam.

1. Fentanyl citrate (sublimaze) is a narcotic analgesic and may be administered via the intramuscular or intravenous route at a standard dosage of 50 µg (0.05 mg/ml). A 100 µg dose of fentanyl is equivalent to 10 mg of morphine or 75 mg of meperidine.
   a. The drug provides analgesia and sedation, but it can also produce respiratory depression and decreased pulmonary exchange, which is treated with naloxone.
   b. Fentanyl can also induce bradycardia, which is treated with atropine. Respiratory depression can outlast the analgesic effects.
   c. Standard doses are 50 µg in normal healthy adults to a total of 2–3 µg/kg for minor surgical procedures; 2–3 µg/kg for children 2–12 years of age; and approximately half the usual adult dose for elderly and debilitated patients.
   d. Onset of action is almost immediate after intravenous administration. The usual duration of action is 30–60 minutes.
   e. Drug side effects can be potentiated with the concurrent use of monoamine oxidase inhibitors, tranquilizers, and paralyzer agents. Teratogenic effects and the possibility of excretion in breast milk are unknown.
2. Midazolam HCl (Versed) is a short-acting benzodiazepine central nervous system depressant that produces amnesia and sedation. The 1 mg/1 ml formulation is recommended.
   a. The drug can produce profound respiratory depression and possible respiratory arrest. Therefore, it must be used in conjunction with continuous monitoring of vital signs.
   b. Initial intravenous administration is 1 mg in a normal healthy adult but should not exceed 2.5 mg over 2 minutes, or a total of 5 mg. At my institution, we reduce the initial dose to half in elderly (>60 years) and debilitated patients, to a total of no more than 3.5 mg.
   c. Onset of action after intramuscular administration takes 15 minutes and duration is 30–60 minutes. Intravenous administration produces sedation in 3–5 minutes. Overdosage can be treated with flumazenil, a specific benzodiazepine-receptor antagonist.
3. The initial loading dose is generally adequate sedation for the entire procedure, which takes approximately 30–45 minutes. Nursing personnel are desirable for patient monitoring. At minimum, a pulse oximeter is necessary to provide data regarding pulse rate and oxygen saturation.

V. Equipment

A. Percutaneous spine biopsy requires either fluoroscopy or CT for accurate needle placement.

1. The advantage of fluoroscopy is that real-time imaging is possible. Thus, fluoroscopy may help reduce the time of the procedure in certain instances. This is especially helpful when biopsying the lower intervertebral lumbar disc spaces such as L4-L5 and L5-S1 levels.

2. With CT the needle is advanced in a non–real-time fashion. Thus, images are obtained, the needle is advanced, and the images are repeated in order to determine needle position.

   a. The advantage of CT is that it allows precise needle placement.

   b. For small focal lesions within vertebral bodies or posterior elements, CT allows more accurate placement of the needle tip.

B. Fluoroscopy

   1. Fluoroscopic-guided spine biopsies are performed with the patient positioned in a posterolateral or paravertebral approach.

      a. The patient is initially in the prone position with the side of the suspected abnormality elevated with a pillow, rolled blanket, or foam wedge.

      b. Positioning can be decided based on imaging findings such as asymmetric disc space narrowing, preferential spread of paraspinal extension of inflammatory process, or asymmetric bony erosion.

   2. The patient's back is prepped and draped in a sterile manner; local, subcutaneous anesthesia is achieved with 1% lidocaine.

   3. The standard needle is a 20 gauge, 5.5-inch spinal needle. Single or biplane fluoroscopic guidance is used for needle visualization.

      a. In the oblique position, the needle is advanced just anterior to the superior facet of the inferior vertebral body (Fig. 7–1). Needle position should be confirmed in both the anteroposterior (AP) and lateral planes.

      b. If the patient complains of radicular pain during advancement of the needle, it can be repositioned in a caudal or cranial direction in order to avoid the nerve.

   4. Aspirates can be performed through the spinal needle by attaching a syringe to the needle hub and gently withdrawing and advancing the needle several millimeters in the disc while applying suction to the syringe. If there is no return of aspirate material, a small amount of saline can be injected and then later aspirated.

C. Computed tomography

   1. The patient is positioned in the prone or decubitus position. A radiopaque grid is placed on the patient's back over the region of interest.

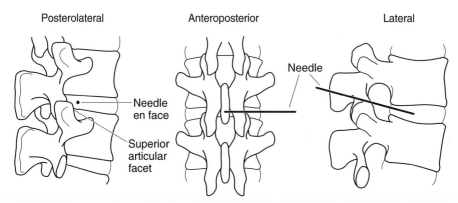

Figure 7-1. Posterolateral approach with fluoroscopic guidance. *Left*, Oblique view with the needle en face with its tip in the mid portion of the disc and anterior to the superior facet of the lower vertebral body. Anteroposterior *(center)* and lateral *(right)* views confirm needle tip position within the middle of the disc. (From Geremia G: Biopsy of Vertebral and Paravertebral Structures with a New Coaxial Needle System. AJNR 13:169–171, 1992.)

2. Slice thickness varies from 3–5 mm. The area is scanned and the axial images are reviewed in order to select the optimal axial section.

   a. The optimal axial section is one in which the lesion is visualized in its largest dimension and a visibly predetermined safe path for the needle can be plotted.

   b. The point for needle entry is determined by two coordinates. The cephalocaudal coordinate is determined by the table position, which is illuminated on the gantry and also on the monitor. The transverse coordinate is determined by the radiopaque grid bars.

3. Most CT scanners include a program known as biopsy mode. This is a feature that allows the operator to move the patient in and out of the CT gantry in order to reposition the needle without repeatedly reprogramming the scanner to obtain images over a selected region of interest.

D. Needles

   1. A standard 20 gauge 5.5-inch spinal needle is used to biopsy an intervertebral disc space under fluoroscopic guidance.

   2. Geremia vertebral needle set. This coaxial needle system is used for precise placement of a biopsy needle following placement of a skinny pilot anesthetic needle. The 16 gauge biopsy needle adequately penetrates the cortical bone of the vertebral body.

   3. MD-Tech biopsy needle. This is a 16 gauge biopsy needle that is 16 cm in length. The tip is designed to penetrate the cortical bone.

   4. A 22 gauge, 25-cm-long cutting needle such as a Westcott is some-

times used coaxially through the 16 gauge needle to obtain multiple cellular specimens for on-site or off-site cytologic examination.

5. Max-Core needle, designed for use in paraspinal soft tissue (Fig. 7–2), is available in several needle gauges, sizes, and lengths. This core needle biopsy device is intended for use in soft tissues such as the paraspinal muscles and adjacent soft tissues. Precaution should be taken so that bone is not struck during needle firing. This could cause the stylet to bend at the specimen notch.

VI. Needle Techniques

A. Tandem needle technique (Fig. 7–3)

1. A skinny 22 gauge needle is placed through the skin to the level of the periosteum of the bone. This is used for selective anesthesia. The position of the needle can be guided with either fluoroscopy or CT.

2. The biopsy needle is positioned parallel and in tandem with the skinny 22 gauge needle. This is advanced in freehand. The biopsy needle should lie parallel with the skinny needle, and the tip of the biopsy needle should approximate that of the skinny needle.

3. The 22 gauge needle is withdrawn and the biopsy needle is rotated and advanced in order to penetrate the cortical bone.

4. This technique depends on the hand-eye coordination of the operator when attempting to approximate the position of the biopsy needle tip near that of the skinny needle tip.

B. Coaxial needle technique (Fig. 7–4)[5]

1. This needle system is provided by Cook Inc (see section V. C.). It begins with a skinny 22 gauge pilot needle that has a removable hub. The pilot needle is advanced to the periosteum of the cortical bone. An anesthetic is delivered to the periosteum. The 22 gauge needle acts as a guide over which the 16 gauge bone biopsy needle is placed.

2. The stylet and hub of the needle are removed and replaced with a hubless stylet that adds support and stiffness to the cannula, which is helpful for advancement of the large-bore 16 gauge needle. Thus, the biopsy needle follows the previously determined safe pathway made by the skinny needle.

3. The biopsy needle tip lies at exactly the same point as that of the skinny needle tip, that is, on the periosteum where the greatest amount of anesthesia was deposited.

Text continued on page 143

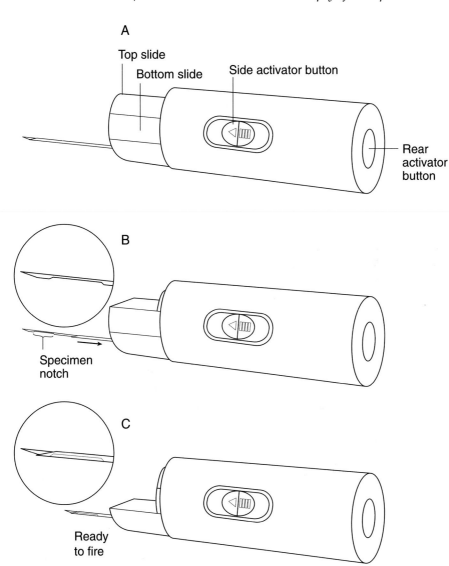

Figure 7–2. Bard Max-Core disposable biopsy instrument. *A,* Biopsy gun prior to energizing (cocking). *B,* The top slide is locked back which pulls back the outer cutting cannula. The inner stylet with its biopsy specimen notch is exposed. *C,* The bottom slide is also locked in place and pulls the stylet into the cannula. The instrument is fully energized (cocked) at this time and is ready to fire. The needle tip should be inserted to the outer margin of the tissue to be biopsied. While maintaining the position of the needle, depress the rear activator button, or push the side activator forward (direction of arrow) in order to advance the stylet and cannula that will obtain the specimen. Remove the needle from the patient and pull back on the top slide to withdraw the cannula and expose the biopsy specimen. The instrument can be re-inserted and re-energized if multiple biopsy specimens are required. (From Geremia G: Biopsy of Vertebral and Paravertebral Structures with a New Coaxial Needle System. AJNR 13:169–171, 1992.)

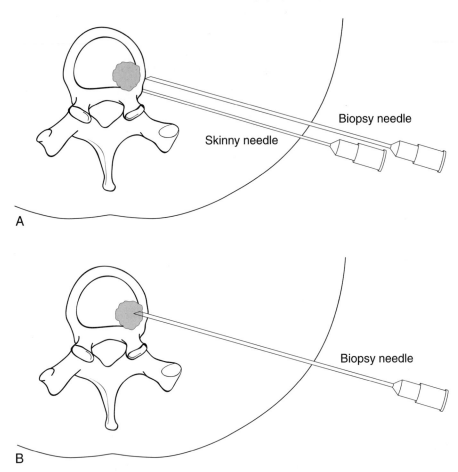

Figure 7–3. Tandem needle technique. *A*, Skinny anesthetic needle is advanced to the periosteum, which is anesthetized with lidocaine. The larger gauge biopsy needle is placed parallel and in tandem with the smaller needle. *B*, The skinny needle is removed and the biopsy needle advanced. (*A* From Geremia G: Biopsy of Vertebral and Paravertebral Structures with a New Coaxial Needle System. AJNR 13:169–171, 1992.)

Figure 7–4. Coaxial needle system technique. *A*, Posterolateral approach to the thoracic vertebral body. The 22 gauge needle is advanced through the skin to the level of the periosteum of the cortical margin of the vertebral body. The periosteum is anesthetized with lidocaine (1%). *B*, The hubbed stylet is removed from the cannula of the 22 gauge needle and is replaced by a hubless stylet. This adds stiffness to the cannula to allow greater ease of tracking of the large biopsy needle. *C*, The 16 gauge biopsy needle tracks coaxially over the 22 gauge hubless stylet and cannula. The large biopsy needle follows the same path as was traveled by the narrow pilot needle. There is no risk of damaging the adjacent lung pleura or other adjacent soft tissues. *D*, The 22 gauge cannula and hubless stylet are removed after the biopsy needle has advanced to the level of the periosteum. The biopsy needle is rotated and advanced through the cortical bone into the medullary cavity of the vertebral body. Aspiration is applied to a syringe attached to the hub of the biopsy needle.

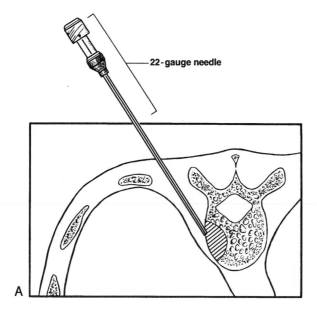

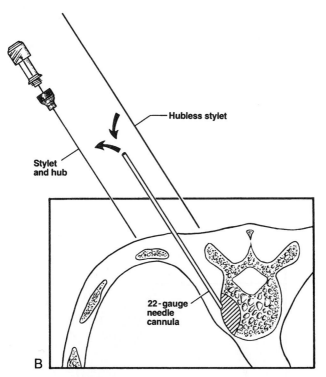

Figure 7–4. *See legend on opposite page*

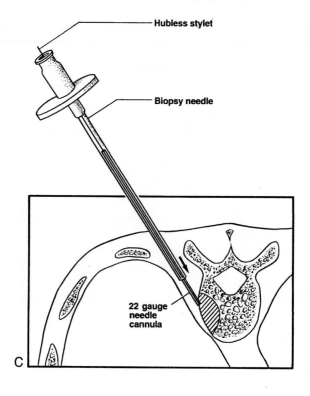

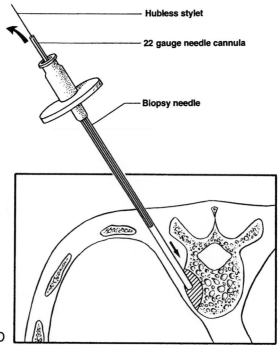

Figure 7–4 *Continued.*

4. After the skinny needle is removed, the biopsy needle is advanced and the specimen is retrieved.

VII. Approaches to the Vertebral Column

A. Cervical spine.[8] The most common approaches used in the cervical region are the anterolateral, lateral, and posterolateral (Fig. 7–5).

1. Anterolateral

   a. With this approach, the anterolateral aspects of the vertebral body and intervertebral disc are accessible. The intervertebral disc is not obstructed by the uncovertebral joint, which is located posterolaterally. The common carotid artery can be manually displaced laterally along with retraction of the sternocleidomastoid muscle.[10]

   b. The needle enters the skin at a point located medial to the anterior margin of the sternocleidomastoid muscle. The common carotid artery and muscle are displaced by retracting them laterally. The biopsy needle is advanced over the ventral surface of the fingers, which are producing retraction of the muscle and underlying vessels. The needle passes between the air space and the common carotid artery.

   c. Needle positioning can be performed with the use of fluoroscopic guidance. Anteroposterior and lateral fluoroscopy should be available to document the exact location of the needle tip.

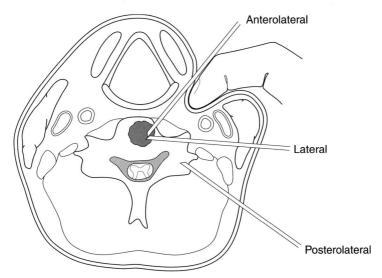

Figure 7–5. Cervical spine approaches. In the anterolateral approach, the sternocleidomastoid muscle and underlying vessels are displaced laterally with manual pressure. Also shown are lateral and posterolateral approaches.

    d. The coaxial system can be helpful in this location by avoiding important vascular and neurogenic structures.

      (1) A 22 gauge pilot needle can be advanced and repositioned until a safe track is determined.

      (2) Once this is established, the 16 gauge biopsy needle can be coaxially placed over the 22 gauge cannula of the needle. This ensures safe passage of the biopsy needle and precludes potential damage to vascular or neurogenic structures.

      (3) Computed tomography ensures accurate placement of the needle tip. Direct visualization of vascular structures is possible with intravenous infusion of contrast agent.

2. Lateral

    a. This approach is valuable for biopsying the anterior body or disc. Intravenous contrast is administered in order to opacify the carotid artery and jugular vein.

    b. The needle enters the skin posterior to the posterior border of the sternocleidomastoid muscle and follows a course posterior to the carotid sheath structures.

    c. For the needle to reach the anterior body or disc, the bony tubercle of the foramen transversarium must be avoided.

3. Posterolateral approach

    a. The posterolateral approach is adequate for biopsying lesions of the posterior elements (e.g., facet joints, lamina, and posterior paraspinal soft tissues). These structures can be approached with near impunity. There are few, if any, important vascular or neurogenic structures within this region.

    b. A coaxial system may be used; however, most of these lesions can be safely accessed with a single needle (noncoaxial).

    c. If a lesion has a large soft tissue component, a 22 gauge biopsy needle may be adequate for obtaining tissue for cytologic examination.

B. Thoracic spine. The common approaches in the thoracic region are the transcostovertebral, transpedicular, and posterolateral (Fig. 7–6).

1. Transcostovertebral[2]

    a. CT guidance and the coaxial needle system are preferred. The patient is placed in the prone or lateral position, and a fine 22 gauge needle is advanced under CT guidance through the anterior part of the transverse process of the vertebra and the posterior part of the neck of the rib.

    b. The tip of the skinny needle is advanced to the lateral cortical

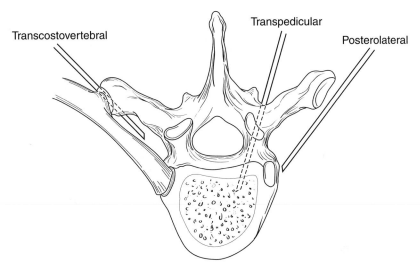

Figure 7–6. Thoracic approaches: transcostovertebral, transpedicular, and posterolateral.

margin of the vertebral body, and the periosteum of the vertebral body is adequately anesthetized with lidocaine.

c. Following placement of the skinny needle, a large biopsy needle can be placed coaxially over the skinny needle. Caudal or cephalic angulation of the needle may be necessary in order to penetrate the interverbral disc space. The advantage of the coaxial approach is the avoidance of any risk to the lung pleura.

d. When the skinny needle has entered the joint space, the remainder of the procedure is safe because the biopsy needle follows the same pathway over the 22 gauge needle.

e. The tubercle of the rib may provide a visual, but not necessarily real, barrier to placement of the needles. If the tubercle acts as an obstruction to the advancement of the 22 gauge needle, minimal cephalad or caudal angulation will redirect the needle so that it slides under the tubercle. Once the tubercle is passed, the tip of the needle enters the joint space and the procedure can be continued without obstruction.

f. The rate-limiting step of this procedure is placement of the skinny needle. Once it is positioned within the joint space the remainder of the procedure advances rapidly.

g. The transcostovertebral approach is safe and provides adequate access to the vertebral body and the intervertebral disc space.

2. Transpedicular[1, 9, 11]

a. The tandem needle technique or the coaxial technique can be used in this approach.

  b. CT guidance is used to document needle position within the lesion. The skinny 22 gauge anesthetic needle is advanced so that its tip lies at the groove between the lateral aspect of the superior articular facet (the mamillary process) and the medial portion of the tranverse process. The periosteum at this site is infiltrated.

  c. The biopsy needle can then be advanced either in a coaxial manner (see section VI. B.) or in tandem (see section VI. A.) to this point on the cortical surface.

  d. Advantages of the transpedicular approach
     (1) The needle track is shorter.
     (2) The transverse process and the mamillary process join at an acute angle and help guide the needle tip toward the pedicle.
     (3) The biopsy needle is perpendicular to the cortex of the bone at the point of entry.
     (4) The cortical bone along the posterior aspect of the pedicle is typically thin.

  e. A possible complication would include an intraspinal hematoma that could compress the spinal cord or the nerve roots.[7]

  f. Biopsy performed by the transpedicular approach must be undertaken with care because the nerve roots lie close to the pedicle. Multiple repeat CT sections are necessary to demonstrate the position of the needle, which should lie within the central portion of the pedicle.

3. Posterolateral

  a. Caution should be taken in order to avoid puncturing the lung pleura. The transcostovertebral approach is preferred.

  b. In order to prevent healthy hard cortical bone tissue from entering the biopsy needle, clogging the lumen, and preventing a biopsy specimen from being taken at the target lesion, the inner stylet (with the MD-Tech biopsy needle) should not be withdrawn until the biopsy needle has passed through the pedicle and has reached a point just before the target site. With the Cook coaxial needle system a 19 gauge needle is locked into the 16 gauge biopsy needle with a Luer-Lok connection (Fig. 7–7).

  c. At this point, the stylet (or a 19 gauge needle within the coaxial system) is withdrawn and the biopsy needle is advanced through the target site, which will obtain tissue only from this region.

  d. The needle is connected to a syringe or to a tube and syringe so that low negative pressure can be applied to aspirate the core.

C. Lumbosacral spine (Fig. 7–8)[6]

  1. Transpedicular—The approach is similar to that in the thoracic spine (see section VII. B.).

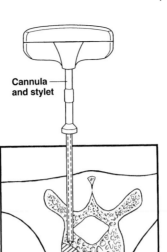

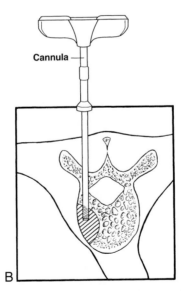

Figure 7–7. *A*, Needle cannula with stylet locked in place is advanced through the cortex and deep within the medullary cavity until the tip abuts the margin of the target lesion. *B*, Remove the stylet and advance only the cannula through the lesion. With the coaxial needle system, a 19 gauge needle included with the system is locked with a Luer-Lok into the 16 gauge biopsy needle and together advanced through the vertebral body to the margin of the target lesion. The 19 gauge needle is removed and only the 16 gauge biopsy needle is advanced into the lesion and the specimen obtained.

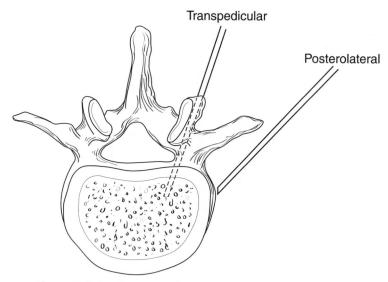

Figure 7-8. Lumbar approaches: transpedicular and posterolateral.

2. Posterolateral

   a. The needle is placed posterolaterally and advanced to the postero-lateral margin of the vertebral body.

      (1) If the path of the needle lies near the foramen, the nerve root may be impinged upon by the needle. In this instance, the patient experiences radicular symptoms, and the needle should be repositioned until radicular pain is no longer elicited.

      (2) Lidocaine is infiltrated into the periosteum of the vertebral body.

      (3) If the coaxial system is used, the large biopsy needle is advanced over the skinny needle cannula. Thus, the ability to elicit radicular symptoms following placement of the skinny needle can act as a functional test.

         a. The skinny 22 gauge needle will not cause permanent damage to vascular structures or nerves; therefore, it can be placed initially to predetermine a safe passage for the biopsy needle.

         b. In the case in which the needle lies near the foramen and radicular symptoms are elicited, the needle tip should be repositioned until the pain is no longer present.

      (4) Localized pain over the site of the needle tip is typical and caused by pain fibers within the periosteum.

b. When the skinny needle no longer elicits radicular symptoms, the pathway is safe for advancement of the biopsy needle.

   (1) The coaxial system is preferred, whereby the biopsy needle follows the same exact predetermined safe pathway that was taken by the skinny needle.

   (2) Also, in the coaxial system the biopsy needle tip lies at the exact same location as the tip of the skinny needle where the anesthesia has been administered in greatest concentration and where the most effective anesthesia occurs.

   (3) The posterolateral approach often requires a long needle to properly traverse the subcutaneous fat and muscles prior to abutting the cortex of the vertebral body.

      a. Ideally, the tip of the needle should lie as perpendicular as possible to the cortical surface of the vertebral body, where it is more likely to penetrate the cortical surface.

      b. When the needle lies more tangential to the outer cortical surface, it is less likely to penetrate and more likely to slide along the outer cortical margin. This could potentially lead to injury to adjacent vessels and cause a paravertebral hematoma.

c. Biopsy under CT guidance is most easily performed when the needle shaft stays within the exact plane of the axial CT slice. Although the L5-S1 intervertebral disc is obliquely angled, it usually can be entered with the gantry at zero degrees. In some instances it may be necessary to traverse bone prior to entering the disc space. This is possible by keeping the stylet locked into the cannula until the disc margin is reached. The stylet is removed and the cannula alone is advanced through the disc. Keeping the stylet within the cannula until the disc margin is approached will prevent traversing bone from plugging the cannula.

d. At times it may be difficult to ascertain the exact cephalocaudal location of the needle tip on the axial images alone.

   (1) The disc space may be difficult to identify in the axial plane when it is narrowed because of partial volume averaging with the adjacent sclerotic vertebral endplates.

   (2) In addition, the needle may add artifact to the axial image.

   (3) The lateral scout image may help to determine the precise cephalocaudal location of the needle tip.[3]

   (4) With the lateral scout view, these problems are eliminated and thus accurate localization is possible.

e. A lateral approach for CT-guided percutaneous biopsy of the lumbar spine has been described.[4] The patient is placed in the decubitus position, which causes anterior displacement of the abdominal viscera, thereby providing a clear view of the lateral aspect of the lumbar spine.

(1) This route provides a wide field for needle insertion, allowing access to the lateral wall of the vertebral bodies and the intervertebral discs.

(2) The perpendicular direction of the needle is easy to maintain, and the needle is a safe distance away from nerve roots, kidneys, the renal pedicle, and large vessels.

(3) This approach should not be used for lesions of the pedicles or vertebral arches or if the forward displacement of abdominal contents is not great enough.

VIII. Post-procedure Care

A. The patient should be closely monitored and observed for at least 2 hours after the procedure.

1. Frequent neurologic checks every 15 minutes for the first hour and then 1 hour later are recommended.

2. Special attention should be given when biopsying lesions near the spinal cord. An emergent CT scan over the biopsy site is recommended if signs suggestive of myelopathy appear.

3. No limitations to activity are necessary unless an underlying debilitating condition exists.

B. Acetaminophen or aspirin is recommended for localized pain at the biopsy site.

C. Outpatients can be discharged 2 hours after the procedure if asymptomatic, and they should be accompanied by another adult.

D. If pain persists or worsens 24 hours after the procedure or unusual symptoms develop, the referring or operating physician should be notified as soon as possible.

E. If symptoms develop that are suggestive of a myelopathy, for example, lower extremity weakness or bowel or bladder incontinence, the operating physician should be notified immediately and the patient admitted to the emergency department.

IX. Procedure Reporting

A. Document discussion of procedure with the patient, including risks.

B. Include pertinent CT findings (e.g., bone destruction, soft tissue mass(es), cord compression, level of lesion).

C. Give details of procedure.
   1. Patient position (e.g., supine, decubitus)
   2. Level of the target lesion
   3. Amount and type of anesthetic agent
   4. Needle system selected and needle approach (e.g., posterolateral, transpedicular)
   5. Type of specimen obtained (e.g., aspirate for cytology, core bone specimen)
   6. Follow-up CT findings over biopsy site (e.g., residual hematoma)
D. List all medications administered and dosages (e.g., Versed 1.0 mg, fentanyl 50 μg).
E. Complications that occurred during or immediately following the biopsy are mentioned.

X. Procedural Coding

CPT Code

A. Biopsy codes
1. Biopsy superficial bone, trocar, or needle (e.g., ileum, sternum, spinous process, ribs)	20225
2. Deep bone (e.g., vertebral body, femur)	20225
3. Biopsy, muscle, percutaneous needle	20206
4. Disc aspirate	62287
B. Supervision and interpretation
1. Fluoroscopic guidance (spine)	76005
2. Computed tomographic guidance	76360

SUGGESTED READING

1. Ashizawa R, Ohtsuka K, Kamimuira M, et al: Percutaneous transpedicular biopsy of thoracic and lumbar vertebrae—method and diagnostic validity. Surg Neurol 52:545–551, 1999.
2. Brugieres P, Gaston A, Heran F, et al: Percutaneous biopsies of the thoracic spine under CT guidance: transcostovertebral approach. J Comput Assist Tomogr 14:446–448, 1998.
3. Coombs R, Ebraheim N, Jackson W: Use of the lateral scout image as an adjunct to computed tomography–guided spinal biopsy. Spine 16:1386–1388, 1991.
4. Garces J, Hidalgo G: Lateral access for CT-guided percutaneous biopsy of the lumbar spine. AJR Am J Roentgenol 174:425–426, 2000.
5. Geremia G, Charletta D, Granato D, et al: Biopsy of vertebral and paravertebral structures with a new coaxial needle system. AJNR Am J Neuroradiol 13:169–171, 1992.
6. Ghelman B, Lospinuso M, Levine D: Percutaneous computed-tomography-guided biopsy of the thoracic and lumbar spine. Spine 16:736–739, 1991.
7. Jamshidi K, Swain W: Bone biopsy with unaltered architecture: a new biopsy device. J Lab Clin Med 77:335–342, 1971.

8. Kattapuram S, Rosenthal D: Percutaneous biopsy of the cervical spine using CT guidance. AJR Am J Roentgenol 149:539–541, 1987.
9. Renfrew D, Whitten C, Wiese J, et al: CT-guided percutaneous transpedicular biopsy of the spine. Radiology 180:574–576, 1991.
10. Tampieri D, Weill A, Melanson D, et al: Percutaneous aspiration biopsy in cervical spine lytic lesions. Neuroradiology 33:43–47, 1991.
11. Ward J, Jeanneret B, Oehlschlegel C, et al: The value of percutaneous transpedicular vertebral bone biopsies examination. Spine 21:2484–2490, 1996.

8

Percutaneous Vertebroplasty

John M. Mathis, M.D., M.Sc.

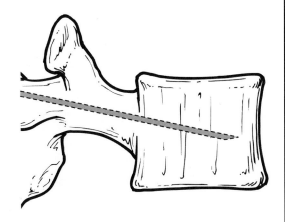

I. Rationale for Procedure and Clinical Indications

A. Percutaneous vertebroplasty (PV) was conceived and started by Herve Deramond in France in 1984. It was first performed for the treatment of pain associated with an aggressive hemangioma of the cervical spine. Deramond treated his first patient by injecting polymethyl methacrylate (PMMA) into a partially destroyed C2 vertebra using fluoroscopic guidance. Pain was permanently relieved in this patient. The procedure was introduced into the United States in 1993 and used primarily for pain associated with osteoporotic compression fractures. Malignant compressions are also amenable to treatment with this procedure.

B. Clinical indications include

1. Painful osteoporotic compression fractures
2. Painful malignant destruction of vertebrae (with or without fracture)
3. Painful aggressive hemangioma or other benign tumors (with or without fracture)
4. Painful vertebral fracture associated with osteonecrosis (Kümmell's disease)

II. Contraindications to Percutaneous Vertebroplasty

A. Asymptomatic, stable fracture
B. Patient rapidly improving on medical therapy
C. Prophylaxis in osteopenic patients with no evidence of new or painful fracture
D. Osteomyelitis or systemic infection
E. Acute traumatic fracture (nonpathologic)
F. Uncorrectable coagulopathy or hemorrhagic diathesis
G. Radicular pain or radiculopathy
H. Tumor extension into the vertebral canal or cord compression
I. Complete vertebral collapse

III. Informed Consent

A. PV is a procedure with potentially severe side effects and complications, and informed consent must be obtained prior to proceeding.
B. The most common complication associated with PV is cement leak. This can be asymptomatic, but it can also cause severe local pain, nerve or cord compression, and pulmonary embolus.
C. PMMA is a foreign body and, while it is inert and unlikely to stimulate an allergic response, infection is a potential complication.

D. Local bleeding at the puncture site can occur.

E. Local trauma due to puncture of adjacent structures or organs (lungs, cord) can occur.

F. Allergic or idiosyncratic reactions to radiographic contrast agent or PMMA are unlikely but possible.

IV. Pertinent Anatomy

A. Transpedicular approach (Fig. 8–1)

   1. The transpedicular approach is the classic method of performing PV. The pedicle offers a safe and easily seen target through which to enter the vertebral body.

   2. The pedicle is a tubular structure and does limit the needle angle and ultimate tip position in the vertebral body. Needle tip position after a transpedicular approach is usually lateral to the midline; therefore, a bipedicular approach is commonly used to get good filling of both hemispheres of the vertebra.

   3. The pedicle can be very small in some individuals (particularly in the high thoracic spine) requiring a reduction in the needle size used (11–13 gauge).

B. Parapedicular (transcostovertebral) approach (Fig. 8–2)

   1. This approach has become increasingly popular in situations in

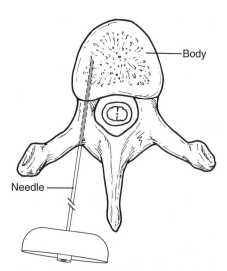

Figure 8–1. Illustration of a trocar-cannula system that has been placed via a transpedicular approach into the vertebral body. Note that the needle tip extends to the anterior portion of the vertebral body.

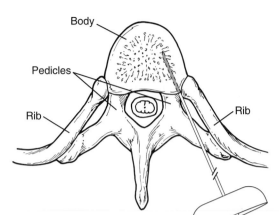

Figure 8–2. The parapedicular (transcostovertebral) approach is shown. The needle is introduced at the level of the pedicle but along its lateral edge rather than through the pedicle.

which the pedicle is not seen well, has been destroyed, or is very small.

2. It does provide an easier trajectory to the center of the vertebra that can facilitate adequate cement filling with one injection.

3. The needle should be placed as close to the lateral edge of the pedicle as possible and at (not below) the level of the pedicle.

4. Although this approach is more appropriate in the thoracic than in the lumbar spine, risk of pneumothorax must be kept in mind.

C. Posterolateral approach

1. Historically used for needle placement in Craig needle biopsies of bone.

2. This approach is similar to the parapedicular trajectory, but the needle enters the vertebra lower (below the level of the pedicle) and puts the exiting nerve root at risk of damage.

3. This approach has no usefulness for PV.

D. Anterolateral approach

1. This approach is reserved for the cervical region.

2. It allows needle entry into the cervical vertebra and avoids the small pedicles in this region.

3. Care must be taken to avoid the carotid-jugular vessels with this approach. Computed tomography (CT) guidance can be helpful to ensure avoidance of these vascular structures.

V. Equipment Requirements

A. Image guidance

 1. Fluoroscopy is the primary imaging method used for performing PV.

 a. It allows real-time needle placement and monitoring of cement injection.

 b. It is readily available in all radiology departments.

 c. Standard, fixed plane fluoroscopy is insufficient for this procedure.

 d. Either a modern single or biplane C-arm fluoroscopy room is necessary to provide adequate visualization.

 e. Biplane fluoroscopy is preferred but not essential for PV.

 2. CT scanning has been used infrequently for needle placement.

 a. CT gives good contrast resolution.

 b. CT is not real time in nature and cannot provide as safe a guidance for needle introduction or cement injection as does fluoroscopy.

 c. Motion is detrimental to a good CT scan, and usually general anesthesia is needed to minimize motion with this modality.

 d. CT is cumbersome, slower, and more expensive to use than fluoroscopy.

B. Needle selection and injection device selection

 1. Numerous manufacturers provide needle systems that are suitable for PV. These devices are usually intended for bone biopsy and consist of an 11-gauge trocar and cannula system.

 2. All of these systems currently come with a fixed handle that can be introduced by direct hand pressure or tapping with a mallet. (The mallet provides good control but produces more pain, and I still introduce the needle by hand.)

 3. Several needle tip geometries are available. The simplest is the bevel tip. The sharp triangular tip provided in the Stryker-Howmedica vertebroplasty kit seems to work best for holding its position in bone and cutting through the cortex.

C. Cement selection

 1. All cements used for PV are some form of PMMA.

 2. No cement is specifically approved for PV at the time of this writing.

 3. The only PMMA that is approved as a structural agent for use in all bone (including the spine) is Simplex-P.

 4. All cements require additional opacifier for visualization with fluoroscopy.

 a. Barium sulfate is the most common opacifier used in PMMAs.

b. Twenty percent–30% of barium sulfate by weight is needed to produce adequate opacification for PV.

c. Barium sulfate must be sterile; sterilization can be accomplished only with radiation or dry heat (steam and ethylene oxide are not adequate).

VI. Sedation and Anesthesia

A. Local anesthesia

1. Injection of local anesthesia is required (unless the patient receives general anesthesia) for PV.

2. The local anesthetic is injected into the skin and subcutaneous needle track and over the periosteum where the needle osteotomy is made to enter the pedicle.

3. Lidocaine produces a burning sensation and may be modified with the addition of bicarbonate and buffered solutions (such as Ringer's solution). These modifications allow local anesthesia without the intense burning found with lidocaine alone.

4. Local anesthetic should be used liberally for patient comfort.

B. Conscious sedation

1. Adjunctive use with local anesthetics

2. Common drugs include fentanyl (Sublimase) and midazolam (Versed).

3. These drugs are titrated according to the patient's needs, body size, age, and medical condition.

C. General anesthesia

1. Rarely needed for routine PV

2. May be indicated in patients who cannot lie prone for the procedure or who have psychological problems that limit cooperation

3. Commonly required if CT is used for needle guidance due to the need for motion control

D. Patient monitoring

1. Physiologic monitoring should include the following:

a. Electrocardiogram

b. Blood pressure

c. Oxygen saturation

E. Nursing support

1. Needed to monitor the patient during the procedure and administer sedation at the direction of the radiologist

2. Postoperative care and observation for signs of complications

3. Follow-up in 24–48 hours to check the patient's response and answer questions. These data are useful for quality assessment as well.

VII. Procedure

A. Antibiotics

1. All patients should receive antibiotics before the procedure.
2. The most commonly employed antibiotic is 1 g of cefazolin given intravenously.
3. Antibiotics in the cement are recommended only in patients who are immunocompromised. When added to the cement, 1.2 g of tobramycin powder is commonly used.

B. Positioning

1. The procedure is performed with the patient prone on the radiographic or operative table.
2. Padding should be added to the table for patient comfort.
3. C-arm boards that allow support and comfortable positioning are recommended.

C. Sterile preparation

1. The area to be treated is prepared in sterile manner per operating room standards.
2. Complete sterile drapes should be applied.
3. All surfaces that come in contact or near contact with the patient should be covered (image intensifiers, and so on).
4. A working table should be set up that is sterile for instruments and cement mixing.
5. Everyone in the room should wear scrub suits, caps, and masks.
6. Room traffic should be minimized.

D. Sedation and anesthesia

1. As described previously (see section VI. B.), conscious sedation is given as needed.
2. Local anesthesia is used for the skin, subcutaneous tissue, and periosteum.

E. Needle placement

1. The trocar-cannula selected is directed through the skin surface to the periosteum of the lamina overlying the pedicle. This is accomplished with image guidance.
2. A small osteotomy is made in the bone, and the needle is advanced through the pedicle into the vertebral body.

3. The tip of the needle should be advanced beyond the midpoint of the vertebral body (as viewed from the lateral projection) (Fig. 8–3).

F. Venography

1. This is used by some physicians to determine the flow of cement

2. In our experience, this procedure is not useful and increases patient radiation, contrast agent exposure, and cost.

3. Venography does not accurately predict cement flow.

4. This step is not needed to safely perform PV.

G. Cement injection

1. The cement is mixed using a vacuum mixing chamber supplied by the cement manufacturer.

2. Sterile barium sulfate is added in sufficient quantity to produce a 25%–30% mix (by weight).

3. Changing the powder-to-liquid ratio leads to structural changes in the cement and should be done cautiously. I do not advise changing these ratios.

4. Chilling the liquid (monomer) before mixing and keeping the mixed cement chilled during the procedure extends the working time of the procedure.

5. Cement is injected with 1-ml syringes. These small syringes allow maximum control of the cement and generate adequate pressure for injection.

6. Cement injections are carefully monitored in real time with fluoroscopy.

7. Vertebral filling is more easily accomplished if one needle is placed in each pedicle before cement mixing and injection.

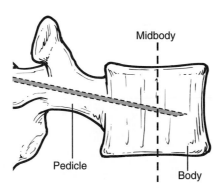

Figure 8–3. Lateral view showing a needle in place via a transpedicular approach. The needle tip extends into the anterior part of the vertebral body.

8. Monitoring in two planes is necessary to ensure that cement does not leak outside the confines of the vertebral body during injection. Cement leaks are an indication for termination of the injection.

9. The lateral projection gives the best view to ensure that cement does not leak into the epidural space or anteriorly into the vena cava.

10. Adequate filling of a vertebra is subjective and varies according to the patient's body size, location in the spine, and amount of compression. Generally, 4–8 ml of cement adequately fills a vertebra (Fig. 8–4).

11. After vertebral filling, the cannulas can be removed. It is common to have rather brisk venous bleeding from the puncture sites. Local pressure for 3–5 minutes is generally sufficient to obtain hemostasis.

VIII. Post-procedure Care

A. The patient is maintained recumbent for 2 hours after the procedure (90% of the cement's ultimate strength is obtained in 1 hour).

B. Betadine ointment is applied to the puncture sites and covered with a sterile bandage.

C. Analgesics are given as needed.

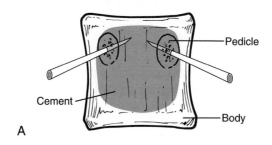

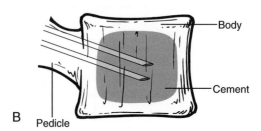

Figure 8–4. *A* and *B*, AP and lateral illustrations show a typical cement distribution during the injection procedure.

D. Vital signs and neurologic evaluations (focused on the lower extremities) are monitored every 15 minutes for the first hour and before discharge.

E. If the monitoring period is uneventful, the patient is discharged to the care of a family member or adult friend who will be available to see him or her home and continue follow-up care for 24 hours.

F. If an increase in pain, significant change in vital signs, or a neurologic change occurs, an immediate evaluation should be started to determine the cause.

    1. A CT scan is useful to determine if there has been leakage of cement outside the vertebra that could cause compression of a nerve or the spinal cord.

    2. Any neurologic change should initiate an immediate surgical consult as well.

    3. Post-procedure pain can be caused by PV. However, prompt evaluation should be performed to ensure that no problem exists that requires intervention.

    4. Post-PV pain may be treated with nonsteroidal anti-inflammatory drugs, analgesics, and local steroid-analgesic injections.

IX. Procedure Reporting

A. Clinical history: This should include a statement about the reason for the procedure such as the etiology of the compression fracture (i.e., osteoporosis), failure of conservative therapy, and diagnostic methods that identified the vertebra chosen for treatment.

B. Antibiotics administered

C. Anesthesia given

D. Vertebra treated

    1. Levels treated

    2. Needle approach

    3. Number of needles placed

    4. Type of cement (including any modifications such as opacifier added)

    5. Amount of cement injected at each level

    6. Any complications experienced

E. Monitoring and follow-up results

X. Procedural Coding

A. Until 2001 there has been no uniform coding for PV in the United States.

B. In 2001, the American College of Radiology developed dedicated CPT codes, as follows:

	CPT Code
1. Vertebroplasty	
a. PV—thoracic	22520
b. PV—lumbar	22521
2. Vertebroplasty supervision and interpretation	
a. Sacroiliac (SI) charge with fluoroscopy guidance	76012
b. Sacroiliac (SI) charge with CT guidance	76013

C. Additional levels are charged.

D. Venography and needle placement are not separate charges.

E. Biopsy can be charged separately for each level where this actually occurs prior to PV.

F. Coding should reflect the method of image guidance (fluoroscopy, CT, and the like).

SUGGESTED READING

1. Barr JD, Barr MS, Lemley TJ, McCann RM: Percutaneous vertebroplasty for pain relief and spine stablization. Spine 25(8):923–928, 2000.
2. Belkoff SM, Maroney M, Fenton DC, Mathis JM: An in vitro biomechanical evaluation of bone cements used in percutaneous vertebroplasty. Bone 25:23S–26S, 1999.
3. Bostrom MP, Lane JM: Future directions. Augmentation of osteoporotic vertebral bodies. Spine (Suppl): 22:38S–42S, 1997.
4. Chiras J, Depriester C, Weill A: Percutaneous vertebral surgery. Technics and indications. J Neuroradiol 24:45–59, 1997.
5. Cooper C, Atkinson EJ, Jacobsen SJ, et al: Population-based study of survival after osteoporotic fractures. Am J Epidemiol 137:1001–1005, 1993.
6. Cooper C, Atkinson EJ, O'Fallon WM, Melton LJ III: Incidence of clinically diagnosed vertebral fractures: a population-based study in Rochester, Minnesota, 1985–1989. J Bone Miner Res 7:221–227, 1992.
7. Cotten A, Boutry N, Cortet B, et al: Percutaneous vertebroplasty: state of the art. Radiographics 18:311–323, 1998.
8. Cotten A, Deramond H, Cortet B: Preoperative percutaneous injection of methyl methacrylate and N-butyl cyanoacrylate in vertebral hemangiomas. AJNR Am J Neuroradiol 17:137–142, 1996.
9. Cotten A, Dewatre F, Cortet B, et al: Percutaneous vertebroplasty for osteolytic metastases and myeloma: effects of the percentage of lesion filling and the leakage of methyl methacrylate at clinical follow-up. Radiology 200:525–530, 1996.
10. Cyteval C, Sarrabere MP, Roux JO, et al: Acute osteoporotic vertebral collapse: open study on percutaneous injection of acrylic surgical cement in 20 patients. AJR Am J Roentgenol 173:1685–1690, 1999.
11. Deramond H, Depriester C, Galibert P, Le Gars D: Percutaneous vertebroplasty with polymethylmethacrylate. Technique, indications, and results. Radiol Clin North Am 36:533–546, 1998.
12. Deramond H, Depriester C, Toussaint P: Vertebroplasty and percutaneous interventional radiology in bone metastases: techniques, indications, contraindications. Bull Cancer Radiother 83:277–282, 1996.

13. Deramond H, Depriester C, Toussaint P, Galibert P: Percutaneous vertebroplasty. Semin Musculoskelet Radiol 1:285–295, 1997.
14. Deramond H, Galibert P, Debussche C, et al: Percutaneous vertebroplasty with methylmethacrylate: technique, method, results [abstract]. Radiology 177P:352, 1990.
15. Galibert P, Deramond H, Rosat P, Le Gars D: Preliminary note on the treatment of vertebral angioma by percutaneous acrylic vertebroplasty. Neurochirurgie 33:166–168, 1987.
16. Jasper LE, Deramond H, Mathis JM, Belkoff SM: The effect of monomer-to-powder ratio on the material properties of cranioplastic. Bone (Suppl):25:27S–29S, 1999.
17. Jasper L, Deramond H, Mathis JM, Belkoff SM: Evaluation of PMMA cements altered for use in vertebroplasty. Presented at the 10th Interdisciplinary Research Conference on Injectible Biomaterials, Amiens, France, March 14–15, 2000.
18. Jensen ME, Evans AJ, Mathis JM, et al: Percutaneous polymethylmethacrylate vertebroplasty in the treatment of osteoporotic vertebral body compression fractures: technical aspects. AJNR Am J Neuroradiol 18:1897–1904, 1997.
19. Kado DM, Browner WS, Palermo L, et al: Vertebral fractures and mortality in older women: a prospective study. Study of Osteoporotic Fractures Research Group. Arch Intern Med 159:1215–1220, 1999:
20. Mathis JM, Eckel TS, Belkoff SM, Deramond H: Percutaneous vertebroplasty: a therapeutic option for pain associated with vertebral compression fracture. J Back Musculoskelet Rehabil 13(1):11–17, 1999.
21. Riggs BL, Melton LJ III: The worldwide problem of osteoporosis: insights afforded by epidemiology. Bone 17:505S–511S, 1995.
22. Tohmeh AG, Mathis JM, Fenton DC, et al: Biomechanical efficacy of unipedicular versus bipedicular vertebroplasty for the management of osteoporotic compression fractures. Spine 24:1772–1776, 1999.
23. Weill A, Chiras J, Simon JM, et al: Spinal metastases: indications for and results of percutaneous injection of acrylic surgical cement. Radiology 199:241–247, 1996.

9

Discography

Douglas Scott Fenton, M.D.
and Leo Frank Czervionke, M.D.

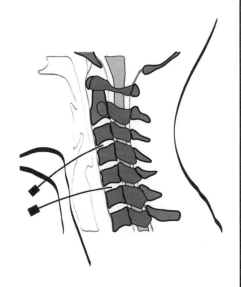

I. Rationale for Procedure and Clinical Indications

A. Introduction

1. Discography is one of the many procedures available to assess a patient's back or neck pain.

2. Magnetic resonance imaging (MRI) is the first imaging study that should be obtained in the setting of acute back pain.

3. In patients with unexplained chronic back pain, discography may provide valuable information regarding a possible discogenic origin of the pain.

   a. Until recently, "discogenic pain" as a cause of significant back pain has not been widely accepted and therefore the role of discography in the past has been controversial.[2, 7, 8, 12]

   b. Although disc morphology may be assessed using radiographs, computed tomography (CT) and MRI, discography is the only imaging procedure for the assessment of back pain that directly correlates the patient's pain response to internal disc morphology.[3, 7]

4. The technique for performing discography has undergone many refinements in the past several decades. The criteria for diagnosing a positive discogram have also changed.

5. In modern discography, a positive pain response is represented as pain that is concordant with the patient's symptoms elicited by a low volume injection (1.5–3.0 ml) that often correlates with radial or concentric tears on postdiscogram radiographs and CT.

B. Discography procedure

1. Discography involves percutaneously placing a needle into a disc, injecting a low volume of contrast agent, and then assessing the patient's immediate pain response.

2. Subsequently, radiographs and post-procedure CT scans are usually obtained to document disc morphology.

3. *The primary value of discography is in the clinical assessment of the patient's pain response and not in the imaging assessment of the disc anatomy.*

C. Discography and MRI

1. MRI is considered the primary screening modality for the evaluation of back pain.

2. Discography is more sensitive than MRI for detection of internal disc disruption including annular fissures (tears).

3. MRI may show areas of T2 signal hyperintensity in the annulus

referred to as "high intensity zones," which have a high correlation with the discogenic pain associated with annular fissures.[1, 11]

4. Approximately 13% of patients with annular fissures visible on MRI are asymptomatic.[7] Before surgical or other disc-related interventions, discography may provide valuable information.

D. Back and neck pain

1. There are many causes of back and neck pain. Often the cause of a patient's back pain is complex and multifactorial.

2. Nerve endings have been demonstrated in the outer one third of the annulus fibrosus, and encapsulated nerve receptors have been identified along the lateral surface of the annulus fibrosus.[2, 3] The posterior longitudinal ligament and ligamentum flavum are also innervated.[2, 3]

3. Pain can often be elicited by injecting contrast into the nucleus pulposus of a morphologically normal or abnormal disc.

   a. It is not important to determine whether or not pain can be elicited. The key factor in diagnosis lies in whether the pain produced by the injection is typical (concordant) or not typical (discordant) of the patient's usual pain.

   b. It is important to localize the level(s) from which the pain is originating.

E. Indications for discography

1. Discography should never be the initial procedure performed for the purpose of diagnosing disc herniation or in the setting of acute back or neck pain. MRI is the procedure of choice for evaluating disc herniation and nerve root involvement in the acute setting.

2. Until recently, discography was primarily performed in preoperative evaluation for the assessment of potential spinal fusion levels.

3. Indications for discography

   a. Evaluation of levels above or below a potential fusion to provide information on whether those levels should be included in or excluded from the fusion

   b. To assess discs at, above, or below an existing fusion in patients with failed back syndrome

   c. To assess back or neck pain in patients with minimal or no findings on imaging studies such as MRI or CT

   d. To determine symptomatic disc levels in patients with multilevel disc abnormalities on imaging studies

   e. A test of exclusion when other tests and therapies have failed to identify the source of back pain

f. Although no longer performed in the United States, chemonucleolysis is still performed elsewhere and requires pre-procedure discography.

g. Pre-procedural evaluation for intradiscal electrothermal annuloplasty (IDET)

   (1) Pre-IDET discography must be performed to confirm that the disc is the source of pain and which levels are symptomatic.

   (2) Pre-IDET discography is also important because it establishes whether there is adequate access to the disc before the IDET procedure, and it also establishes the size and shape of the nucleus pulposus, which is useful in determining proper needle placement during IDET.

   (3) Pre-IDET discography and post-discography CT provide important information about the internal architecture of the disc and establish not only if there is a radial tear but also the location and direction of the tear. The direction of the tear may prove to be useful information in establishing the side of the approach to the disc, because it has been observed that it is easier to cross a radial tear with the IDET thermal catheter at an acute angle to the tear as opposed to an obtuse angle.

II. Contraindications

A. Coagulopathy (international normalized ratio [INR] >1.5 or platelets <50,000/mm³)

B. Pregnancy (to prevent fetal radiation exposure)

C. Either systemic or local infection involving the skin of the puncture site(s)

D. Severe allergy to any of the medications used in the procedure

E. A previously operated-on disc may or may not yield reliable information and should be carefully scrutinized if discography is performed.

F. The theoretical risk of causing or aggravating myelopathy from slight enlargement of the disc during discography in patients with spinal cord compromise at the level of the proposed discography

G. An extensive, solid posterior bone fusion may not allow for percutaneous disc access

III. Informed Consent

A. The procedure is explained to the patient.

B. The risks and potential complications are explained to the patient.[4, 6, 14]

1. Bleeding
2. Infection (specifically disc infection and the potential for vertebral osteomyelitis)
3. Thecal sac puncture and headache
4. Allergic reactions pertaining to the medications used in the procedures
5. The risk of pneumothorax for thoracic discography
6. The potential for a clinically significant hemorrhage into the spinal canal and its complications, especially for cervical discography
7. Vasovagal reactions, especially for cervical discography

C. Signed consent is then obtained.

IV. Anatomic Considerations

A. A thorough understanding of the important anatomic landmarks is important prior to performing discography.
B. Lumbar discography
   1. The standard discographic approach is obtained by placing the patient prone and angulating the fluoroscopic beam so that the lumbar disc is punctured posteriorly from a 45-degree left posterior oblique (LPO) or right posterior oblique (RPO) approach.
   2. Access to a given lumbar disc is optimally visualized when the superior articular facet of the vertebral body below is positioned midway between the anterior and posterior disc margins, and the x-ray beam is angulated slightly caudad or cephalad so that the superior endplate margins of the caudad vertebral body superimpose (Fig. 9–1).
   3. Using this technique, the exiting nerve from the upper level is located well above the anticipated needle path, allowing safe entry into the midportion of the disc.
   4. Entry into the L5-S1 disc requires a modification of this approach.
      a. The iliac crest in the oblique position often impedes needle access to the central portion of the disc.
         (1) It may be necessary to angle the beam ±10–15 degrees from the standard 45-degree LPO or RPO angle.
         (2) It may also be necessary to direct the x-ray beam in a cephalocaudad direction.
         (3) The L5-S1 skin puncture is actually slightly more cranial than the L4-L5 skin puncture (Fig. 9–2).
      b. When the beam is properly positioned, a small triangular-shaped

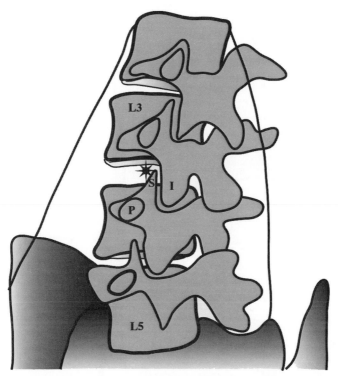

Figure 9-1. Drawing of fluoroscopic image of lumbar spine with patient in prone RAO position (relative to table top), with the facet joint at L3-4 positioned midway along the AP diameter of the disc. The needle target zone (*) is located just anterior to the superior articular process of L4. Note that the superior endplates of L4 superimpose. L3 = 3rd lumbar vertebral body, L5 = 5th lumbar vertebral body, P = pedicle of L4, S = superior articular process of L4, I = inferior articular process of L3.

pathway can be seen on the fluoroscopic image allowing safe needle passage into the center of the L5-S1 disc.

    (1) This triangle is formed by the superior articular facet of S1 medially, the iliac crest laterally, and the L5 vertebral body superiorly (Fig. 9–3).

    (2) Occasionally, no suitable passage into the L5-S1 disc can be located. In this situation, a midline transthecal approach to the L5-S1 disc should be considered, although this approach is rarely necessary.

C. Thoracic discography

    1. The disc is approached with the patient prone and angulating the fluoroscopic beam 35–40 degree in the LPO or RPO projections.

    2. Whether the thoracic discogram is performed using CT or fluoroscopy, the needle is placed just lateral to the superior articulating

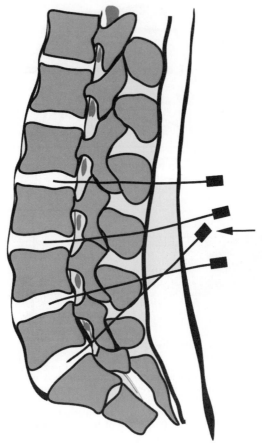

Figure 9–2. Drawing of fluoroscopic image of lumbar spine as viewed in lateral projection with discographic needles placed with their tips in the center of the lower four lumbar intervertebral discs. Note that the L5 needle *(arrow)* punctures the back skin surface superior to the puncture site of L4 and that there is significant craniocaudad angulation of the needle to enter the L5-S1 disc.

process of the caudal vertebra and medial to the head of the ipsilateral articulating rib (Fig. 9–4). Understanding this anatomic relationship allows contrast deposition into the disc slightly off center at the junction of the middle and outer one third of the disc.

a. If one attempts to puncture the thoracic disc medial to the ipsilateral articulating processes, that is, an interlaminar puncture, the spinal cord is in jeopardy.

b. If the thoracic disc is approached more laterally, the lung may be punctured and this can result in pneumothorax.

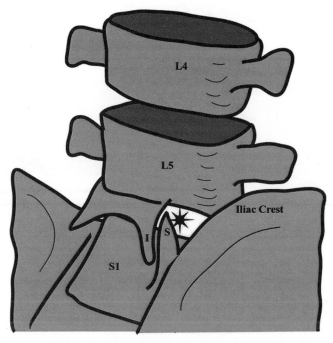

Figure 9–3. Drawing of fluoroscopic image at lumbosacral junction with patient in LAO position. Looking along the craniocaudad path of the needle tract at the needle entry point (*) into the L5-S1 disc. Note the characteristic triangular-shaped window formed by the superior articular process (S) of S1 medially, L5 vertebral body superiorly, and iliac crest laterally. L4 = 4th lumbar vertebral body, S1 = 1st sacral vertebral body, I = inferior articular process of L5.

D. Cervical discography

　1. The disc cannot be approached posteriorly because of the spinal cord.

　2. Posterolaterally, access to the cervical disc is impeded by the vertebral artery and uncinate process.

　3. The cervical airway prevents access into the cervical disc from a direct anterior approach.

　4. Therefore, the cervical disc is approached anterolaterally by manually displacing the carotid artery, internal jugular vein, and sternocleidomastoid muscle (Fig. 9–5).

V. Equipment Requirements for All Spinal Levels

A. Procedural

　1. 22 gauge, 6-inch (or 3.5-inch) spinal needle (one for each disc level, lumbar or thoracic)

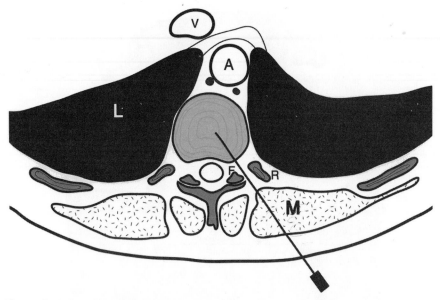

Figure 9–4. Drawing of axial CT scan at the lower thoracic spine level showing the needle path for the thoracic CT-guided discographic approach. The needle passes obliquely through the paraspinal muscles (M) through a small window formed by the facets (F) medially and the head of the rib (R) laterally. L = lung, A = aorta, V = inferior vena cava.

2. 25 gauge, 3.5-inch spinal needle (one for each cervical or thoracic disc level)

3. C-arm fluoroscopy

4. 3-ml Luer-Lok syringe (one for each disc level)

5. 12-ml control syringe with 25 gauge, 1.5-inch needle for local anesthesia

6. Lead apron and sterile gown

B. Medications

1. Non-ionic myelographic contrast 300 mgI/ml

2. Lidocaine MPF (methylparaben free), 1%

3. Bupivacaine hydrochloride, 0.25% or 0.5% MPF (Sensorcaine MPF)

4. Cefazolin (Ancef), 1 g intravenous piggyback

5. Cefazolin (Ancef), 10 mg/5 ml normal saline

6. Clindamycin, 600 mg intravenous piggyback

7. Clindamycin, 6 mg/5 ml normal saline

8. Atropine (cervical discography)

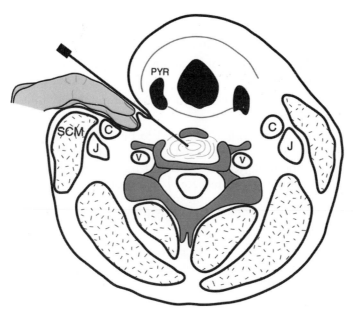

Figure 9–5. Drawing of an axial image of cervical spine at the C4-5 level showing the manual compression technique for cervical discography. Carotid artery (C) and internal jugular vein (J) are displaced laterally and posteriorly by the index and third fingers, allowing needle placement into the cervical disc using anterolateral approach. V = vertebral artery, PYR = pyriform sinus.

C. Incidentals
  1. Povidone-iodine (Betadine) scrub
  2. Alcohol scrub
  3. Sterile drapes
  4. Sterile gauze
  5. Adhesive bandages
  6. Hats, masks, and sterile gloves
D. Precautions
  1. Preservative-free medications
    a. MPF means methylparaben free.
    b. The MPF form is preferable for use in spine intervention procedures because steroid is often given at the same time.
    c. Many steroid suspensions when mixed with certain preservatives may cause flocculation of the steroid.[5]
    d. Some preservatives, if they are inadvertently injected intrathecally, can cause arachnoiditis.

2. Discitis prevention

   a. Discitis is a known complication of discography.

   b. It is recommended that an antibiotic be given to decrease the risk of infection.

   c. 1 g of intravenous cefazolin is given routinely within 1 hour of the procedure.

   d. 1 mg of cefazolin is also added to the injection mixture for each disc. Each 3-ml syringe used for disc injection should contain 2.3 ml of non-ionic iodinated myelographic contrast and 0.5 ml of cefazolin (10 mg/5 ml) for a total volume of 2.8 ml. This will leave enough space in the syringe to draw back on the needle to be sure you are not in a vascular structure prior to injecting the mixture.

   e. If the patient has a known cephalosporin or penicillin allergy, 600 mg of clindamycin can be given intravenously with 0.6 mg (6 mg/5 ml) added to each disc injection syringe.

   f. If the patient has a known allergy to iodine, gadolinium (MRI contrast) or sterile saline can be substituted.

VI. Conscious Intravenous Sedation and Patient Monitoring

A. Patient sedation is usually not required for discography.

B. If conscious intravenous sedation is required, a mild sedative and analgesic are given.

   1. 1–2 mg midazolam

   2. 100–150 μg fentanyl

   3. These can be administered during the procedure to make the patient more comfortable; however, the patient must not be sedated to the point of being unable to give reliable information about the quality and distribution of the pain.

C. Monitoring of electrocardiogram, pulse oximetry, and blood pressure should be performed if sedation is used. Monitoring can be performed during the procedure by a nurse, physician, or physician assistant.

VII. Procedure

A. Preparation

   1. Discography is usually performed on an outpatient basis.

   2. All patients are instructed to withhold their usual pain medications on the day of the procedure so that the discographic evaluation will be more valid.

3. Patients are also required not to drive for the remainder of the day because sedation may be given.

4. An intravenous antibiotic, usually cefazolin, is given within 1 hour prior to the procedure.

B. Lumbar discography

1. Patient positioning

   a. The patient is placed prone on the fluoroscopy table.

   b. The less symptomatic side is elevated on a wedge or pillow 10–15 degrees to facilitate needle puncture. Disc puncture should be performed contralateral to the patient's more symptomatic side to minimize the chance of a false-positive or misleading pain response.

   c. The patient's lower back is prepared and draped in sterile fashion.

2. C-arm positioning

   a. The disc to be punctured is placed in the center of the field of view.

   b. The C-arm is rotated contralateral to the symptomatic side until the apex of the superior articulating process (ear of the "Scottie dog") of the caudal vertebral body is midway between the anterior and posterior aspects of its vertebral body. Also, the superior endplates of the caudal vertebral body at the level of interest should superimpose (see Fig. 8–1).

   c. Significant caudal angulation often is required at L5-S1 to optimally visualize the correct pathway (see Fig. 8–3).

3. Procedure

   a. Lidocaine, 1%–2%, is then given along the expected path of the needle track.

   b. The spinal needle is then inserted parallel to the x-ray beam and advanced using intermittent fluoroscopy.

   c. The needle should remain just ventrolateral to the superior articulating process and midway between the vertebral endplates (see Fig. 8–1).

      (1) With use of this approach, the possibility of contacting the exiting nerve root or passing through any vital structures is minimal.

      (2) This needle pathway will allow needle tip placement into the center of the nucleus.

      (3) The patient often describes a brief sharp pain as the needle passes through the disc's outer fibers (Sharpey's fibers).

      (4) One can feel the change in sensation as the needle passes

from the firm, gritty-feeling outer annular fibers into the less resistant, smooth nucleus.

d. The needle needs to be positioned with its tip in the middle third of the disc in both anteroposterior and lateral planes to ensure intranuclear contrast placement (see Fig. 8–2).

   (1) If the needle is too far lateral, ventral, or posterior, an annular deposition of contrast agent may result.

   (2) An annular injection may give a false-positive or misleading pain response.

e. The needles should be placed in all discs being evaluated prior to the injection of any contrast material. (*Editor's Note*: It should be noted that some operators perform discography one disc at a time.) It is recommended that at least one "normal" or control level be injected to serve as a baseline for the patient's pain tolerance.

f. Once the needles are all in position, they are injected one at a time without the patient knowing which disc is being injected.

   (1) The order of injection should be from the least symptomatic (control) level to the suspected most symptomatic level.

   (2) Slow disc injection is performed under lateral fluoroscopy and should be terminated if and when firm resistance is met.

      (a) If there is firm resistance at the beginning of the injection, this may indicate an annular injection (Fig. 9–6).

      (b) The contrast needs to be evaluated in both AP and lateral views to make sure the contrast is located central (intranuclear) versus peripheral (annular).

      (c) Some authors believe that a manometer should be used during disc injection and that the disc should be injected until either pain is elicited or a specific atmospheric pressure (4–5 atmospheres or 120–150 mm Hg) is reached.[10]

      (d) The annulus is not considered intact if resistance to the injection is not encountered.

      (e) A normal lumbar disc can accommodate 1.5–3.0 ml of fluid.

   (3) The needles remain in place until all levels have been injected.

4. Patient questioning

   a. Pain location

   b. Pain intensity (on a scale of 0–10) elicited by injection

   c. Any significant body posturing or facial grimacing during the injection

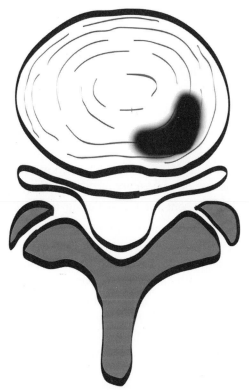

Figure 9–6. Illustration of intra-annular contrast deposition within a lumbar intervertebral disc on post-discogram CT scan. Needle tip was not advanced far enough into the disc center.

    d. Is the pain typical of the usual pain in distribution and quality?

    e. The volume of the mixture instilled into the disc.

    f. Whether or not there was a firm end point (intact annulus)

       (1) It is important to instill an adequate amount of contrast agent into the disc in order to distend the annulus in an attempt to provoke pain sensation.

       (2) If severe pain is elicited at low volumes, then that injection is terminated.

       (3) These subjective findings should be recorded at the time of the procedure by either a technologist or a nurse and should be noted in the physician's dictation.

 5. Intradiscal anesthetic

    a. At concordant pain levels, 0.5 ml of local anesthetic can be instilled through the needle.

    b. The patient's pain is often alleviated immediately, which further substantiates that the particular disc is at least part, if not all, of the origin of their discogenic pain.

   c. Anesthetic injection may also serve to diminish a false-positive response at other disc levels due to residual pain from injections at other levels.

6. After all intended disc levels are assessed, the needles are removed.

7. AP and lateral radiographic images of all injected disc levels are obtained.

8. The patient's back is then cleansed to remove the antiseptic agent, and small adhesive bandages are applied to the puncture sites.

9. The patient is then sent for CT scanning for additional imaging of the injected disc levels.

C. Thoracic discography

1. Thoracic disc degeneration is a frequent cause of annular tears that can be associated with clinically significant pain and disability.

2. Patients may complain not only of midback and chest wall pain but also of visceral, abdominal, and upper lumbar pain.

3. Thoracic discography must be approached with caution given the possibility of causing a pneumothorax or puncturing the thecal sac.

4. Procedure

   a. Fluoroscopically guided technique

     (1) Thoracic discography can be performed safely fluoroscopically, similar to lumbar discography.

     (2) Twenty-five gauge, 3.5-inch spinal needles are preferred because they are of smaller diameter, of shorter length, and their use causes less trauma, because the depths of thoracic discs are less than those of lumbar discs.

     (3) Unlike in lumbar discography, it may be difficult to visualize the thoracic superior articulating process. However, the superior articulating process always projects above the pedicle, which is easily visualized.

     (4) In thoracic discography, the superior articulating process is not positioned to project over the center of the disc as it is in lumbar discography. Instead, the approach is steeper, and the superior articulating process is positioned approximately 30%–40% of the distance across the AP diameter of the vertebral body. This technique allows safe insertion of the needle tip into the disc at the junction of the middle and outer one third of the disc. Any more angulation of the C-arm would cause the costovertebral junction to obstruct the entry point.

(5) One must always be careful to keep the needle tip just lateral to the superior articulating facet and medial to the costovertebral junction (Fig. 9–7). This will ensure that the pleura is not punctured laterally and that the spinal canal is not entered medially.

b. CT-guided technique

(1) As in the fluoroscopic technique, the needle is placed between the superior articulating process and the costovertebral junction (see Fig. 9–4).

(2) The CT scanner gantry optimally should have no cranial or caudal angulation.

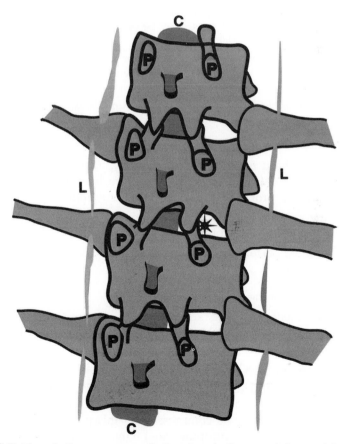

Figure 9–7. Thoracic discogram approach. Drawing of a fluoroscopic image of thoracic spine with the patient in LAO position. Oblique view of the spine from the back shows the target entry site (*) into the disc located medial to the head of the ipsilateral rib and just lateral to the superior articular process of the vertebral body below. The articular processes in the thoracic region are often difficult to visualize at fluoroscopy, but the entry site is in the portion of the disc just superior to the pedicle (P) of the vertebral body below. C = spinal cord, L = lung.

(3) CT scanning is performed using spiral technique at 3-mm-slice thickness.

(4) The gantry is not angled, so the entire disc may not be seen on a single image. One should choose the slice position at which the posterior aspect of the disc is best visualized.

(5) When the posterolateral annulus is contacted by the needle, at the junction of the middle and outer one third of the thoracic disc, the needle tip is usually directed toward the center of the disc when advanced.

(6) The final positions of the needles can be confirmed with a single spiral acquisition through the discs followed by re-formatted sagittal and/or axial images parallel to the disc. These final CT images can also be used to assess for pneumo-thorax, or a chest x-ray may be obtained if a pneumothorax oc-curs.

(7) CT scanning does not allow for the real-time morphologic evaluation of the disc, as one would see using fluoroscopy. However, it still provides all other essential information; *most importantly, the clinician can determine the patient's pain response.*

D. Cervical discography

1. Necessity of cervical discography

   a. Besides the usual risks of discography, a cervical discogram has the added risk of a clinically significant hemorrhage and/or my-elopathy if proper technique is not strictly followed.

   b. Some authors have reported a complication rate as high as 13% for cervical discography.[4]

   c. One must perform a risk-benefit analysis prior to performing this procedure.

2. Patient positioning

   a. The patient is placed supine on the fluoroscopy table with a cushion placed under his or her shoulders to slightly hyperextend the neck.

   b. The patient's neck is prepared and draped in sterile fashion.

   c. During cervical discography, the carotid artery is manually dis-placed to allow safe needle passage into the cervical disc. As the carotid body may be compressed by this procedure, administra-tion of intravenous atropine, 0.6–1.0 mg, is recommended to mini-mize the possibility of a vasovagal response.

   d. As in lumbar discography, the cervical disc should ideally be punctured on the side opposite that of the patient's symptoms.

      (1) This may be technically difficult.

(2) Many discographers believe that a right-sided approach should be used for right-handed discographers, and left-handed discographers should use a left-sided approach.

3. C-arm positioning

a. The fluoroscope is placed in the AP position, and cranial or caudal angulation of the tube is used to optimally visualize the disc space.

b. The spinal needle can be placed parallel to the disc space and viewed fluoroscopically to guide the level of needle insertion along the medial border of the sternocleidomastoid muscle.

4. Procedure

a. Needle puncture should be made between the carotid sheath and the airway.

b. The carotid pulse at the disc level is palpated with the index and middle fingers, and the carotid sheath structures are displaced posterolaterally (see Fig. 9–5).

c. Local anesthesia is then given along the expected needle track.

d. Skin puncture with a 25-gauge, 3.5-inch spinal needle is then performed at a 30–40 degree angle in front of the fingertips used to displace the carotid sheath structures.

e. The needle is then positioned with its tip in the center of the disc, and placement is confirmed with AP and lateral fluoroscopy (Fig. 9–8).

f. Needle injection, patient questioning, and fluoroscopic imaging are performed identical to lumbar discography.

g. The normal cervical disc holds only 0.5–1.0 ml of fluid.

(1) Care should be taken not to overfill the cervical disc.

(2) Venous filling during cervical intradiscal injection is often observed but is of no clinical significance.

h. Post-discography CT scans are then done.

E. Post-procedure imaging

1. Post-discography CT scanning is more sensitive to changes in disc morphology due to internal disc disruption than discography radiographs.

2. CT scanning can be performed in one of two ways:

a. Continuous spiral CT

(1) The patient is placed supine.

(2) Imaging is performed with spiral technique to include all injected discs in one acquisition.

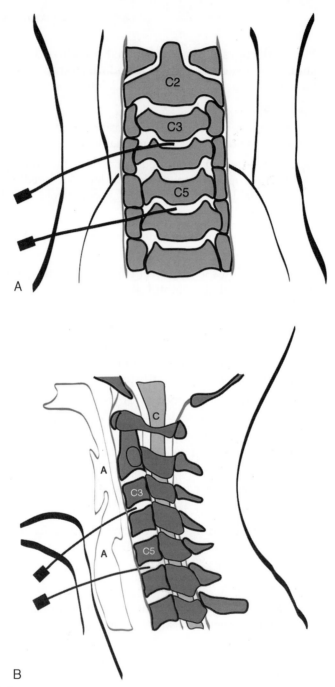

Figure 9–8. *A* and *B*, Cervical discography. *A* depicts an AP fluoroscopic image of the cervical spine showing needle placement in the C3-4 and C5-6 intervertebral discs following anterolateral approach. *B* shows good needle position in the two cervical intervertebral discs on the lateral fluoroscopic projection. Proper needle positioning for cervical, thoracic, and lumbar discography should always be confirmed fluoroscopically in two projections. C = spinal cord, A = airway.

(3) Axial reformatted images parallel to each disc from the pedicle above to the pedicle below can then be obtained, as well as sagittal and coronal reformatted images.

b. Standard CT scanning of discs

(1) Each disc level is imaged separately.

(2) The CT gantry is angled to each disc.

(3) Scanning is performed from pedicle to pedicle.

3. Slice thickness for either method should be 3 mm for lumbar or thoracic discograms and 1 mm for cervical discograms.

VIII. Post-procedure Care

A. The patient should be observed for 2 hours after the discogram.

B. The patient can be allowed to sit in a reclining lounge chair.

C. If there is significant pain or if sedation was administered, the patient should be placed on bed rest.

D. Evaluation of blood pressure, pulse, and respiration is performed every 30 minutes.

E. The patient should be discharged to the care of a responsible adult.

F. The patient is requested not to drive for the remainder of the day, especially if sedation was given.

G. A prescription for a nonrenewable narcotic and/or a muscle relaxant is given to the patient.

H. A discharge sheet should be given to the patient outlining:

1. The procedure performed and at what levels

2. Post-procedure symptoms that usually resolve within 1 week

a. Localized pain at the needle puncture site(s)

b. Possible increased back stiffness

c. Deep back pain

3. Treatment for mild post-procedure symptoms

a. Rest for 3–4 days

b. Avoid prolonged standing or sitting upright

c. Apply ice to the area that hurts

4. Evaluate for signs and symptoms of possible disc infection.

a. Fever

b. Chills

c. Back pain that is different from the patient's usual back pain

5. Evaluate for more serious symptoms.

   a. Stiff neck
   b. Difficulty walking
   c. Bowel or bladder abnormalities
  6. Provide the physician's name and contact number in case any problems arise secondary to the procedure.

IX. Procedure Reporting

A. Clinical assessment of the pain response
   1. The discogram report summarizes all information obtained from the discogram and post-discogram CT.
   2. Each level is reported separately containing information about
      a. The patient's pain response (severity, location, and similarity to his or her usual pain). *The pain response is the most important aspect of discography.*
      b. The amount of the injection mixture instilled into the nucleus
      c. Presence or absence of pain relief following local anesthetic injection and disc morphology
   3. One method to classify the pain response is as follows:
      a. Absence of pain
      b. Pain dissimilar to usual pain (discordant)
      c. Pain identical to part or all of the usual pain (concordant)
B. Imaging assessment
   1. Disc morphology is assessed from the radiographic images and CT scans.
   2. The "normal" disc has various appearances.
      a. Discogram (Fig. 9–9).
         (1) A "cottonball" appearance in younger patients[13]
         (2) A "hamburger bun" appearance[13]
      b. On CT imaging, the normal disc commonly has an oval appearance that remains within the center of the disc (Fig. 9–10).
   3. Annular injection
      a. If needle placement is not in the middle third of the disc in both AP and lateral projections, an annular injection may occur.
      b. An annular injection appears as a collection of contrast agent within the annulus along the periphery of the disc (see Figs. 9–6 and 9–9).
      c. The clinician must be aware of an annular injection because it can lead to a false-positive pain response.

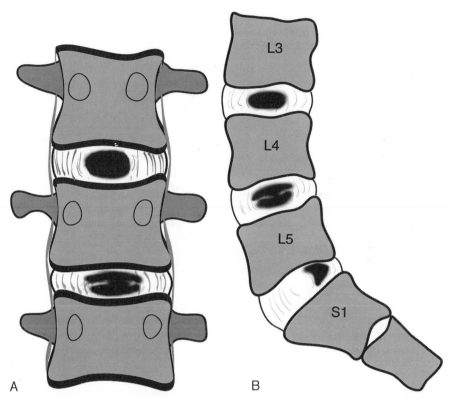

A

B

Figure 9–9. *A* and *B,* Discographic appearance of normal intervertebral discs. *A* is of an AP radiographic image of lumbar spine following discography. Contrast collection has typical oval "cottonball" configuration of a normal intervertebral disc in a young person. The contrast collection in the lower disc space is the bilaminar, or "hamburger bun," appearance of the normal mature disc. In lateral radiographic projection *(B),* the normal "cottonball" configuration of the contrast deposit is seen in the L3-4 disc, the "hamburger bun" appearance appearance of the normal mature disc is seen in the L4-5 disc, and a posterior intra-annular contrast deposit is shown in the L5-S1 disc.

4. Annular tears

a. May be related to trauma, disc degeneration, or the aging process.

b. Three main types (Fig. 9–11)

(1) *Radial tears* extend outward from the disc center toward the disc periphery causing a fissure perpendicular to the circumferential annular fibers.

(2) *Circumferential tears* involve the interlamellar fibrous bridges that normally connect the circumferential annular fibers and cause the lamellar fibers to separate resulting in annular laxity and generalized disc bulging.

(3) *Transverse tears* are usually small tears that occur when the

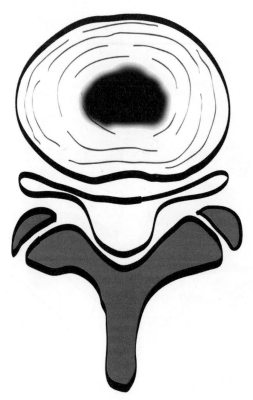

Figure 9–10. Drawing of a post-discogram axial CT scan of a normal disc. The intranuclear contrast deposit has an oval configuration.

annular fibers are torn from the vertebral body at the ring apophysis. Such tears may be related to vertebral osteophyte formation.

c. The radial tear is considered to be the most important factor in discogenic pain. The Modified Dallas Discogram Scale[1, 9] is the standard used for describing the radiographic or CT discographic appearance of annular disruptions of the cervical, thoracic, and lumbar discs.

(1) A normal disc is considered Grade 0 (Fig. 9–12; see also Figs. 9–9 and 9–10).

(2) The radial tear may be confined to the inner third of the annulus (Grade 1) which fluoroscopically may look like a small tail extending from the central nucleus but not reaching the disc margin. (Fig. 9–13; see also Fig. 9–12).

(3) Grade 2 tears (Fig. 9–14; see also Fig. 9–12) extend to the middle one third of the annulus.

Text continued on page 195

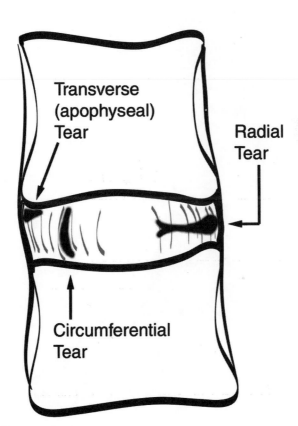

Figure 9–11. Drawing showing AP of lateral anatomic view of intervertebral disc morphology illustrating the three basic types of annular tears (fissures).

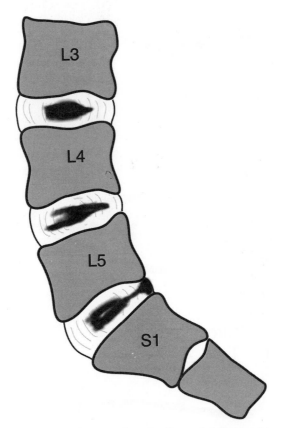

Figure 9-12. Drawing of a lumbar spine lateral radiograph following 3-level lumbar discography. Illustrated are a Grade 1 radial tear in the L3-4 disc posteriorly, Grade 2 anterior and posterior radial tears in the L4-5 disc, and a Grade 3 posterior radial tear in the L5-S1. In the Grade 3 tear, the contrast extends from the disc center to the outermost margin of the annulus posteriorly.

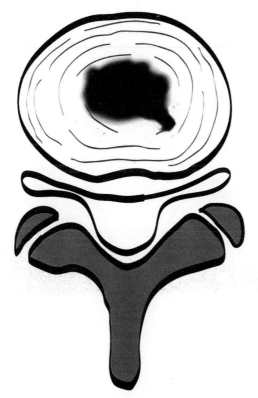

Figure 9–13. Drawing of a post-discogram axial CT scan image of a posterolateral Grade 1 radial tear involving the inner third of the annulus.

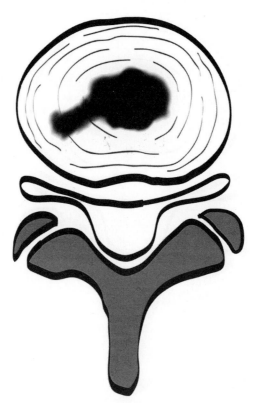

Figure 9-14. Drawing of a post-discogram axial CT scan image of posterolateral Grade 2 radial tear that extends to the middle third of the annulus.

(4) Grade 3 radial tears extend to involve the outer annular fibers (Fig. 9–15; see also Fig. 9–12).

(5) A tear that extends to the outer annulus and covers more than 30 degrees of the disc circumference is considered a Grade 4 tear (Fig. 9–16).

(6) A tear that extends through all layers of the outer annulus and extends or extravasates into the epidural space is termed a Grade 5 tear (Figs. 9–17 and 9–18).

(7) A thin line of contrast agent seen extending from the central nucleus on a 45-degree angle toward the posterolateral margin of the disc may represent the spinal needle track and is not a tear. This must be correlated with the true path of the needle.

5. The aging disc

a. Complex tears of the disc are more often seen.

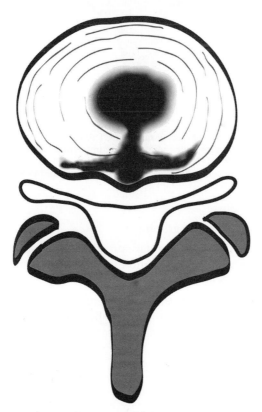

Figure 9–15. Drawing of a post-discogram axial CT scan image of a midline posterior Grade 3 radial tear that involves all layers of the annulus. Grade 3 tears are often associated with a focal protusion of the disc margin, as shown here.

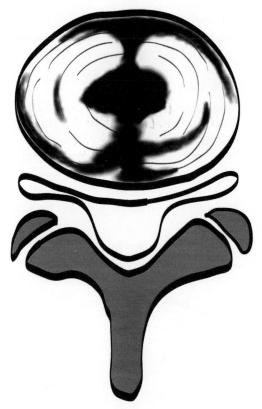

Figure 9–16. Drawing of a post-discogram axial CT scan image of a Grade 4 annular tear. In this type, the annular fissures have radial and circumferential components and the annular tears involve more than 30% of the disc circumference. The outer disc contour bulges diffusely in all directions. Diffuse, severely degenerated discs often fall into this category.

    b. Appearance at discography

        (1) Usually diffuse irregular spread of contrast is seen throughout the entire disc compatible with full-thickness tears with or without epidural spread (see Fig. 9–18).

        (2) Epidural spread can be subligamentous or through the ligament, can be seen to spread above or below the disc injected, and may enter the neural foramen.

X. Procedural Coding

CPT Code

A. Lumbar spine

    1. Discography, lumbar, radiologic supervision and interpretation   72295

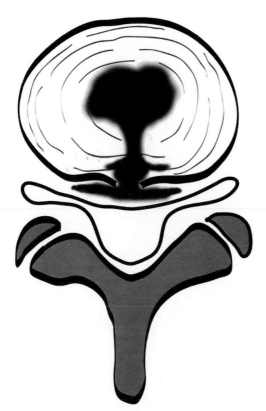

Figure 9–17. Drawing of a post-discogram axial CT scan image of radial tear that has extended through all layers of the posterior annulus in the midline posteriorly. Contrast material extravasates into the ventral epidural space compatible with a Grade 5 radial tear.

    2. Injection procedure for discography, each level;   62290
       lumbar

    3. Computed axial tomography, lumbar spine; with-   72131
       out contrast material

B. Cervical or thoracic spine

    1. Discography, cervical or thoracic, radiologic super-   72285
       vision and interpretation

    2. Injection procedure for discography, each level; cer-   62291
       vical or thoracic

    3. Computed axial tomography, *cervical* spine; without   72125
       contrast material

    4. Computed axial tomography, *thoracic* spine; with-   72128
       out contrast material

C. Cervical, thoracic, or lumbar spine

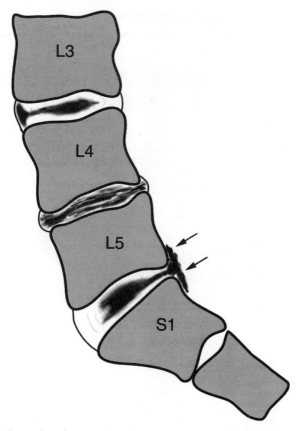

Figure 9–18. Spectrum of severe disc degeneration. Drawing of a post-discogram lateral radiograph depicting an anterior Grade 3 tear of the L3-4 disc. At the L4-5 level, the discographic contrast permeates throughout the entire disc. This is the most common pattern observed in the severely degenerated disc. Note the outer annulus is bulging but is intact. At the L5-S1 level, a Grade 5 annular tear with extravasation *(arrows)* into the ventral epidural space is illustrated.

1. Coronal, sagittal, multiplanar, oblique, 3-dimen-　76375
   sional and/or holographic reconstruction of computed tomography, magnetic resonance, or other
   tomographic modality
2. Can add this code if performing orthogonal re-　76375
   formatted images from the axial CT images

SUGGESTED READING

1. Aprill CN, Bogduk N: High-intensity zone: a diagnostic sign of painful lumbar disc on magnetic resonance imaging. Br J Radiol 65:361, 1992.

2. Bogduk N: The innervation of the lumbar spine. Spine 8:286, 1983.
3. Bogduk N, Windsor M, Inglis A: The innervation of the cervical intervertebral discs. Spine 13:2, 1988.
4. Connor PM, Darden BV: Cervical discography complications and clinical efficacy. Spine 18(14):2035, 1993.
5. *CPT 2000.* Chicago, CPT Intellectual Property Services, American Medical Association.
6. Fraser RD, Osti OL, Vernon-Roberts B: Discitis after discography. J Bone Joint Surg Br 69:31, 1987.
7. Guyer RD, Ohnmeiss DD: Contemporary concepts in spine care lumbar discography. Position statement from the North American Spine Society Diagnostic and Therapeutic Committee. Spine 20:2048, 1995.
8. Holt EP: The question of lumbar discography. J Bone Joint Surg Am 50:720, 1968.
9. Sachs BL, Vanharanta H, Spivey MA, et al: Dallas discogram description: a new classification of CT/discography in low back disorders. Spine 12:287, 1987.
10. Schellhas KP: Discography. Neuroimaging Clin N Am 10:579, 2000.
11. Schellhas KP, Pollei SR, Gundry CR, Heithoff KB: Lumbar disc high-intensity zone. Spine 21:79, 1996.
12. Simmons JW, Aprill CN, Dwyer AP, Brodsky AE: A reassessment of Holt's data on: "The question of lumbar discography." Clin Orthop 237:120, 1988.
13. Tehranzadeh J: Discography 2000. Radiol Clin North Am 36:463, 1998.
14. Zeidman SM, Thompson K, Ducker TB: Complications of cervical discography: analysis of 4400 diagnostic disc injections. Neurosurgery 37:414, 1995.

10

Automated Percutaneous Lumbar Discectomy

Wendell A. Gibby, M.D.

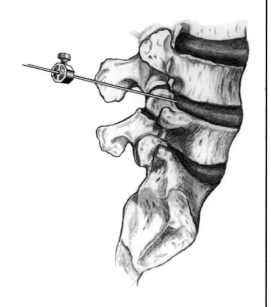

10

Automated Percutaneous Lumbar Discectomy

Gerald A. Grubb, MD

I. Rationale for Procedure and Clinical Indications

A. Herniated lumbar disc disease is one of many etiologies for low back pain and may be a major cause of morbidity and disability. Since Mixter and Barr first reported successful resection of a herniated disc in 1934, controversy surrounding the surgical management of disc disease has persisted. If lumbar disc disease is responsible for pain, reported success rates for simple discectomy and partial laminectomy have ranged between 80% and 95%. Surgery is a major traumatic event to the lumbar spine and adjacent soft tissue, and complication rates vary from less than 1% to 10%[3, 4] (Table 10–1).

B. The failed back syndrome (FBS) is characterized by intractable pain and functional deterioration after spine surgery; it occurs in up to 10% of cases.[5] Since the 1960s, progress improvements in operative techniques using smaller and less invasive procedures have yielded fewer long-term complications. Since the advent of magnetic resonance imaging (MRI) and discography, more precise attribution of pain symptoms to disc origins has been possible. However, the ultimate goal of disc treatment has been to resect or diminish disc herniation through less invasive means to reduce potential complications.

C. Automated lumbar percutaneous discectomy, which is less invasive than surgical discectomy, was first reported by Onik et al. in 1985.[6] This procedure was a major advance over earlier attempts at percutaneous disc removal performed manually with instruments. It accomplished the goal of internal decompression of the intervertebral disc with the least disruption of surrounding tissues.

D. The automated percutaneous discectomy probe uses a reciprocating cutting port with attached vacuum, facilitating removal of nuclear mate-

---

Table 10–1

COMPLICATIONS OF SURGERY

---

1. Epidural, subdural, or paraspinous hemorrhage
2. Abscess and infection, including discitis or osteomyelitis
3. Recurrent or residual disc herniation
4. Paraspinous muscle denervation
5. Facet joint destabilization
6. Neurologic injury with nerve root avulsion or transection
7. Vascular injury
8. CSF fluid leak or pseudomeningocele formation
9. Visceral or ureteral injuries
10. Sexual dysfunction
11. Complications related to surgery and general anesthesia, including deep venous thrombosis, pulmonary emboli, pressure injuries to the eyes, genitalia, and peripheral nerves
12. Death

rial and, more importantly, decreasing the cannula size to a needle-like 2 mm diameter.

E. Hundreds of thousands of patients have had this procedure and numerous clinical studies have indicated that it is safe and efficacious in selected patients.[7-12] Success rates, however, have varied widely depending on the clinician ranging between 50% and 90%.[13] Patient selection, therefore, is crucial in the use of this technology.

F. This technique has several advantages over other percutaneous disc treatment strategies.

   1. Chymopapain, a proteolytic enzyme, can involve rare but potentially devastating complications of anaphylaxis and transverse myelitis.

   2. Percutaneous laser discectomy is harder to control and can result in endplate injuries caused by excessive thermal energy deposition.

   3. With automated percutaneous discectomy, once the procedure is terminated, no further disc removal occurs.

G. The success of the procedure relies on the decompression of a contained disc herniation, protrusion, or bulge, which is believed to be symptomatic on the basis of diagnostic studies. Therefore, the outer annulus must be at least partially intact.

H. Patients who are candidates for percutaneous discectomy tend to be those classified in the less severe spectrum of surgical disc disease.[13, 15] It is precisely this population that is most likely to respond to conservative treatment. Therefore, an extended course of physical therapy should be the first line of therapy. An escalating treatment strategy is initiated, beginning with the most conservative treatment first, as shown in Figure 10–1.

I. The best candidates have the following characteristics:

   1. Young
   2. Athletic
   3. Single-level disc herniation, bulge, or protrusion that is symptomatic.
   4. Contained far lateral disc herniation (the nucleotome passes directly through the herniation site in this case)
   5. Leg pain greater than back pain
   6. The disc herniation is coplanar with the disc
   7. By MRI criteria, the disc is contained
   8. The disc is pressurize-able at discography (a small amount of epidural leakage is acceptable)
   9. The herniation segment of the disc fills during discography
   10. Pain is reproduced at discography

J. Other potential usages:

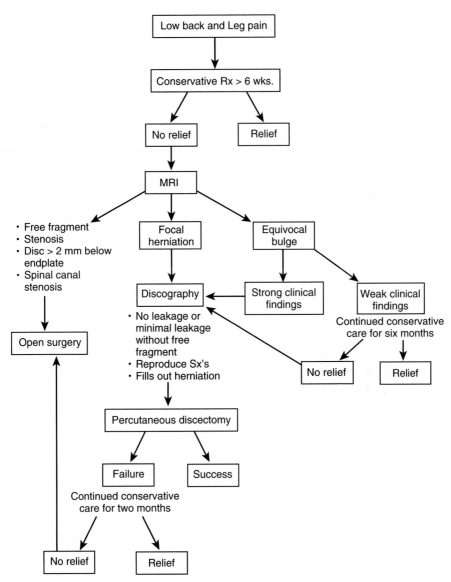

Figure 10–1. Flowchart for percutaneous discectomy patients. (From Zimmerman RA, Gibby WA, Carmody RF: Neuroimaging: Clinical and Physical Principles, New York, Springer-Verlag, Inc., 2000, p. 1489.)

1. Previous open surgery and reherniation (success rates of up to 70% have been reported)[14]
2. For the diagnosis and treatment of discitis

II. Contraindications

A. Lack of adequate conservative treatment
B. Sequestered disc fragment
C. Significant degenerative disease
D. Vacuum disc phenomenon
E. Spondylitic disease
F. Neuroforaminal or spinal canal stenosis
G. Segmental instability
H. Nonsymptomatic disc margin abnormalities
I. Nonconcordant pain production on discography

III. Patient Work-up and Informed Consent

A. Each patient should undergo a thorough history and physical, correlating clinical symptoms with imaging findings. A large percentage of the population has asymptomatic disc herniations. Operating on these patients will do no good. Nerve root compression and the somatomal distribution of pain should be correlated. Pain diagrams are especially useful (Fig. 10–2).
B. Questions to be asked during history include:
   1. Duration of pain? Its severity on a scale of 1–10? The back and leg pain should be rated independently.
   2. Has the patient tried conservative treatments? If so, which? Did they help?
   3. Is the pain getting better or worse?
   4. Which imaging tests have been performed?
   5. Which types of activities make the pain better or worse?
   6. Are secondary gain factors present; e.g., litigation, pending worker's compensation claims, or drug-seeking behavior?
   7. Does the patient have a psychiatric history or history of drug abuse?
   8. What is the patient's occupation?
   9. Does the patient smoke? (Smoking correlates strongly with poor healing.)
C. Physical examination

PAIN DIAGRAM

Patient's Name _____

Date _____

Please shade in the area of pain, numbness, and/or tingling:

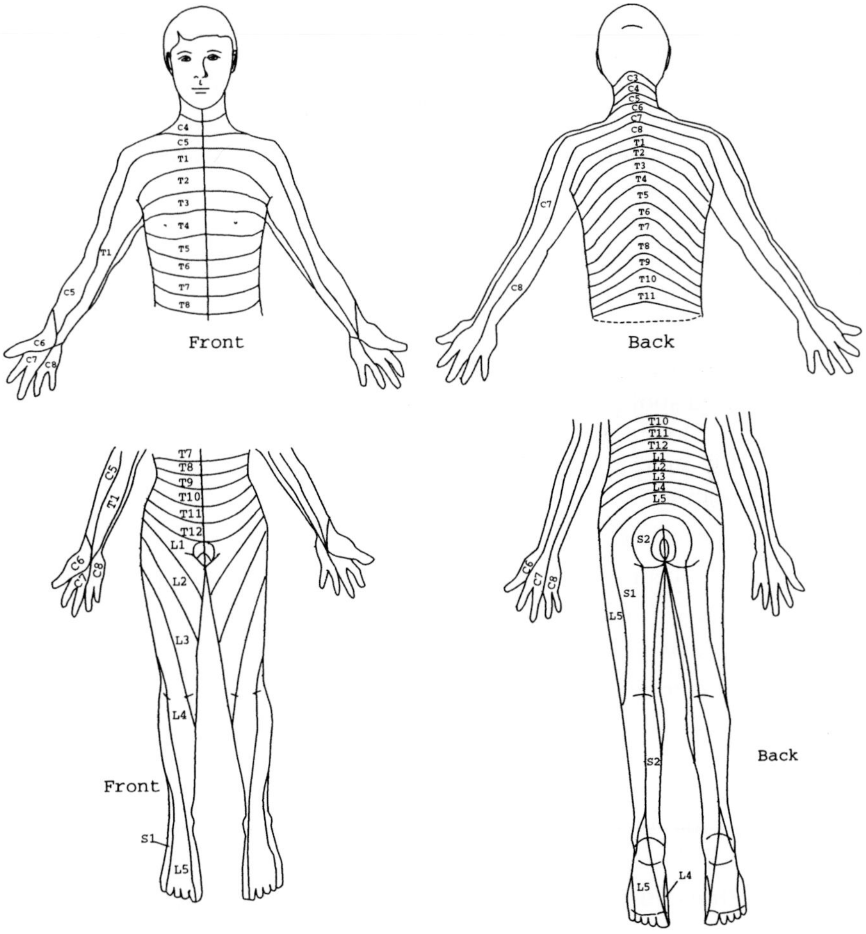

Figure 10–2. Pain diagram.

1. Look for the following:
   a. Radiculopathy
   b. Positive straight leg raising sign
   c. Asymmetric reflexes
   d. Muscle weakness
   e. Gait disturbance
2. Be aware of discordant physical findings, such as bowel or bladder dysfunction, which may point to a more centrally located lesion.

D. Imaging work-up

1. The most common cause of failure has been the presence of a free or sequestered fragment. By means of superior soft tissue contrast and multiplanar capabilities, MRI can greatly facilitate patient selection.

2. Look for integrity of the posterior longitudinal ligament on sagittal images. Discs with a morphologic appearance that are less likely to respond include:
   a. Discs that extend significantly above or below the endplate. I use 3 mm as the cutoff.
   b. Pinched-off discs
   c. A mushroom-type disc that represents an extruded, nonsequestered subligamentous disc herniation still contained by the posterior longitudinal ligament. Figure 10–3 demonstrates types of disc morphology that are not appropriate for percutaneous discectomy.

E. Informed consent

1. As in any surgical procedure, informed consent is mandatory.
2. The most common complication is discitis; it may occur in up to 0.2% of patients. Prophylactic antibiotics should be used.
3. Rarer complications include reflex sympathetic dystrophy, hemorrhage, and neurologic injury.
4. The risks should be kept in perspective. No deaths have been reported. At least the risks are of an order of magnitude less than those for open back surgery, and the risk of the procedure is less than that of a barium enema.
5. A sample informed consent form is shown in Figure 10–4.

IV. Pertinent Anatomy

A. Lumbar disc

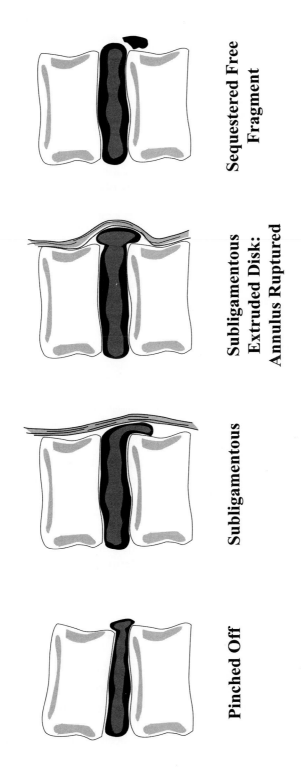

Pinched Off **Subligamentous** **Subligamentous Extruded Disk: Annulus Ruptured** **Sequestered Free Fragment**

Types of discs not appropriate for percutaneous discectomy.

Figure 10-3. Types of discs not appropriate for percutaneous discectomy. (From Zimmerman RA, Gibby WA, Carmody RF: Neuroimaging: Clinical and Physical Principles. New York, Springer-Verlag, Inc., 2000, p. 1489.)

209

INFORMED CONSENT

AM

Date: _____   Time: _____ PM

1. I authorize the performance upon _____
of a PERCUTANEOUS DISCECTOMY to be performed under the direction of

    Dr. _____ .
    (Name of Physician)

2. I consent to the performance of operations and procedures in addition to or different from those now contemplated whether or not arising from presently unforeseen conditions, which the above named physician or his associates or assistants may consider necessary or advisable in the course of the operation.

3. I consent to the administration of such general, spinal, or local anesthetics as may be considered necessary or advisable by the physician responsible for this service.

4. I consent to the disposal by hospital authorities of any tissues or parts which may be removed.

5. The nature and purpose of the operation, possible alternative methods of treatment, the risks involved, and the possibility of complication have been explained to me. No guarantee or assurance has been given by anyone as to the results that may be obtained.

    Signed: _____
    (Patient or person authorized to consent for patient)

    Relationship of person giving
    authorization if not signed by patient: _____

Witness: _____

Figure 10–4. Sample informed consent form.

1. The lumbar disc consists of outer annular layers and the inner nucleus pulposus. In children, the nucleus pulposus and annulus can be distinguished on MRI.[15] However, with aging the highly gelatinous nucleus becomes more fibrocartilaginous, with an increase in collagen content.[16]

2. The nucleus in adults has a physical consistency comparable to that of crabmeat. It is located slightly posterior to the midline of the vertebral body (Fig. 10–5).

3. The outer one third of the annulus contains nocioceptor pain fibers, which can be a source of both low back pain and radicular pain. The inner annulus and nucleus are not innervated.

B. Cartilaginous endcap of the vertebral body

1. The vertebral body endplate serves as a vital conduit for nutrition to the disc, as the normal disc is not vascularized.

2. Damage to the endplate can cause damage to the disc. During surgical discectomy, curettage of disc material can result in damage to the cartilaginous endplates. This has been theorized by some to be a source of continued low back pain.

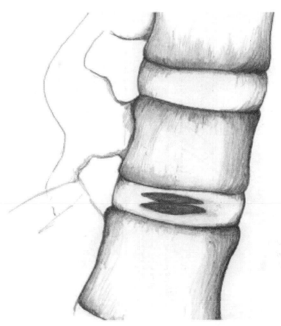

Figure 10–5. AP lateral view of a normal disc. Nucleus is located slightly posterior to the midline of the vertebral body.

3. The automated percutaneous discectomy probe has a blunt tip that does not allow curettage or injury to the cartilaginous endplate.

4. Because the percutaneous discectomy mechanism relies on aspiration for removal of disc material, discs that are highly desiccated (i.e., those in older patients, especially with vacuum phenomenon) are less likely to respond.

5. Hydration of the disc just prior to the procedure via discography is a helpful adjuvant to increasing disc removal yield.

C. Nerve roots

1. The nerve roots exit the dural sac just above the level of the disc beneath the pedicles and extend laterally across the posterior lateral margin of the vertebral body (Fig. 10–6).

2. A knowledge of this anatomy allows a trajectory through which the percutaneous discectomy probe can be safely passed.

D. The inner pedicular line demarcates the position of the dural sac. When the trocar of the procedure contacts the posterior disc margin on the lateral view, it should be in the center of the pedicle on the AP view. If it is medial to the pedicle, then injury to the dural sac may occur.

E. Retroperitoneum: Rarely, patients can have retroperitoneal extension of

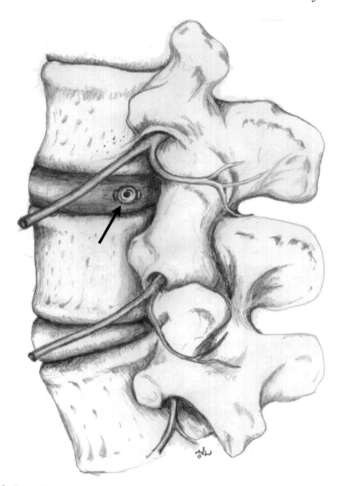

Figure 10–6. Oblique lateral view of the lumbar discs, showing the location of where the needle can pass in order to avoid the nerve root.

colon or other areas of the bowel. It is appropriate to review cross-sectional imaging studies prior to the procedure to ensure that from a paraspinous approach no bowel area is in the anticipated trajectory of the trocar.

V. Equipment Requirements

A. Standard x-ray suite or operating suite with a C-arm (preferably an interventional suite with a rotating C-arm)

B. Automated percutaneous discectomy machine (Surgical Dynamics)

1. Several probe sizes are available. The 2-mm probe is adequate for most cases.

2. Occasionally in young patients with large amounts of hydrophilic disc (not at the L5-S1 level), a 2.5-mm probe is used because disc can be more rapidly removed and is less likely to clog the nucleotome.

C. Discography is performed with a 20 or 22 gauge 15- to 20-cm needle.

D. Non-ionic contrast material at 200 mg/ml is injected. If excessively dense contrast agent is injected (i.e., 350 mg/ml), subsequent trocar placement may be more difficult to see under fluoroscopy.

E. A 10-ml control syringe is utilized for injection. I prefer Merit Medical.

F. Nitrogen tank with pressure regulator.

VI. Sedation

A. Conscious sedation is a vital aspect of the safety of this procedure. With the patient conscious, he or she can inform the operator immediately if nerve root contact is made; the needle can be redirected and nerve injury avoided.

B. Do not perform this procedure with the patient under general anesthesia.

C. Sedation is titrated according to the size and age of the patient. Typically I begin with 3 mg of Versed intravenously and 50 mg Demerol intravenously.

D. Appropriate monitoring of patients is essential, including blood pressure, heart rate, and oxygen saturation.

VII. Procedure

A. Pre-procedure setup:

1. An intravenous line is started. The patient receives a prophylactic dose of 1 g IV of a broad-spectrum antibiotic. (I use Claforan.)

2. Strict surgical asepsis is followed.

   a. The room is prepared as if a pacemaker were to be inserted.

   b. Nurses and radiographic technologists are trained in OR surgical technique by OR scrub nurses.

   c. Band bags are placed over image intensifiers and x-ray tubes, and a full surgical drape is placed over the patient.

B. Trocar placement

1. The patient is placed in the lateral decubitus position. The approach for percutaneous discectomy is paraspinous; it can be performed in

either the prone or lateral decubitus position. I prefer the lateral decubitus position because:

a. On patients with large, protuberant abdomens, image quality is improved in the lateral position, as the mass of the abdomen falls away from the spine.

b. By placing several towels beneath the patient, the spine can be "opened up" (Fig. 10–7).

2. With the C-arm in the AP projection, the patient is placed in a true lateral position by observing the location of the posterior spinous processes relative to the pedicles.

3. The fluoroscope is then moved into a lateral position, and a line parallel to the disc spaces is drawn on the patient's skin to mark the expected trajectory of the trocar into the disc space.

4. A needle is then used to infiltrate the skin and deep fascial tissues with 1% lidocaine, approximately 10–15 cm lateral to the midline. The approach to the disc should be at about a 45-degree angle.

5. The flex trocar provided in the nucleotome kit is passed through a small skin nick created with a No. 11 surgical blade under fluoroscopic control toward the disc.

a. The trocar should contact the disc on the lateral view when the AP view projects midway between the pedicle (Fig. 10–8).

b. If the needle is medial to the inner pedicular line on the AP view there is a chance of passing through the thecal sac (Fig. 10–9). The needle must be withdrawn and redirected slightly more ventrally and laterally.

c. If the needle is placed too far anteriorly or peripherally, the trocar will be in the outer layers of the nucleus, not in the nucleus pulposus (Fig. 10–10).

d. If the needle is too far superior or too far lateral, the exiting nerve root may be impinged upon (Fig. 10–11). The needle should be withdrawn and placed more inferiorly and medially.

e. An anterior trocar placement is not acceptable because the goal of the procedure is to aspirate as much nuclear material as possible and as close to the disc herniation as possible.

f. The trocar in its final position should be located centrally on the AP view and slightly posterior to midline in the lateral view (Fig. 10–12).

6. L5-S1 challenges

a. Patients with high iliac crests and/or large transverse processes at L5 can present difficulty.

b. An AP pelvis film can be useful for pre-operative planning at

Text continued on page 219

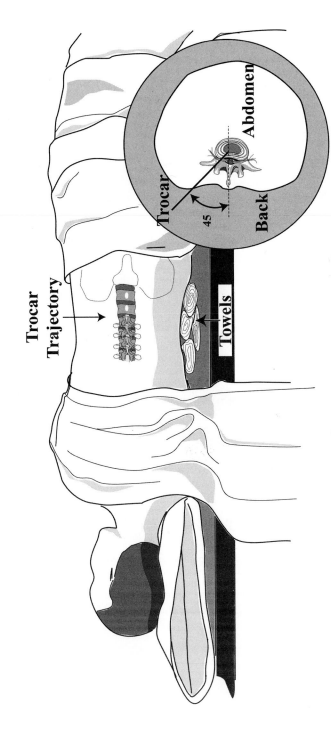

Figure 10-7. Lateral decubitus patient position. The patient has rolled-up towels placed underneath to "open up" the disc space. (From Zimmerman RA, Gibby WA, Carmody RF: Neuroimaging: Clinical and Physical Principles. New York, Springer-Verlag, Inc., 2000, p. 1441.)

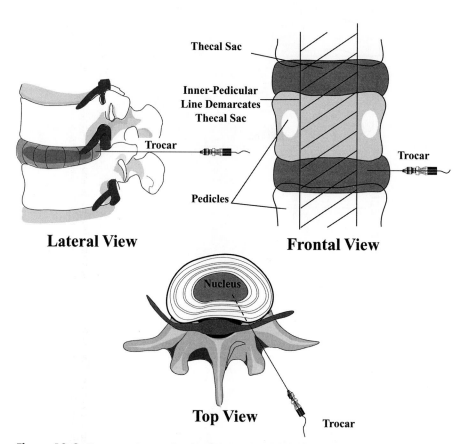

Figure 10–8. Correct trajectory for the discography needle before entering the disc. On the lateral view the needle is touching the posterior margin of the disc. On the AP view the needle lies just medial to the inner pedicular line, which demarcates the thecal sac. This will give a correct trajectory into the center of the nucleus. (From Zimmerman RA, Gibby WA, Carmody RF: Neuroimaging: Clinical and Physical Principles. New York, Springer-Verlag, Inc., 2000, p. 1441.)

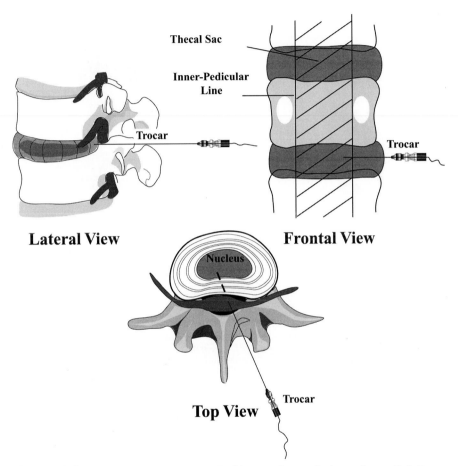

Figure 10–9. Incorrect needle trajectory. In this case the needle is too far medial; it may traverse the thecal sac. On the lateral fluorobeam, the needle contacts the posterior margin of the disc. However, on an AP view, the needle lies medial to inner pedicular line. Thus, the needle is at risk for traversing the thecal sac. (From Zimmerman RA, Gibby WA, Carmody RF: Neuroimaging: Clinical and Physical Principles. New York, Springer-Verlag, Inc., 2000, p. 1442.)

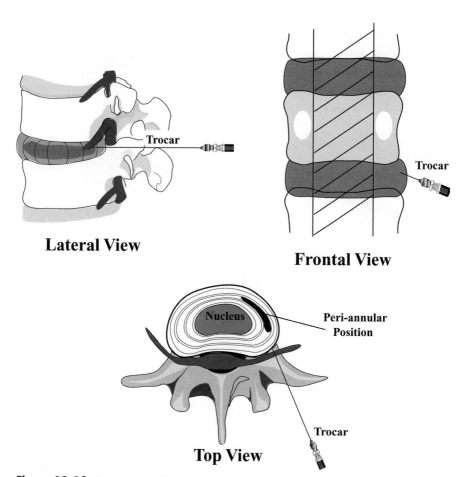

Figure 10–10. Incorrect needle trajectory. The needle is positioned too far laterally. Even though the needle contacts the disc on the lateral view, it is well lateral to the pedicles on the AP view. Such a trajectory will result in a periannular position. It also risks contacting the nerve root and eliciting direct radicular pain. (From Zimmerman RA, Gibby WA, Carmody RF: Neuroimaging: Clinical and Physical Principles. New York, Springer-Verlag, Inc., 2000, p. 1443.)

NEEDLE PLACEMENT

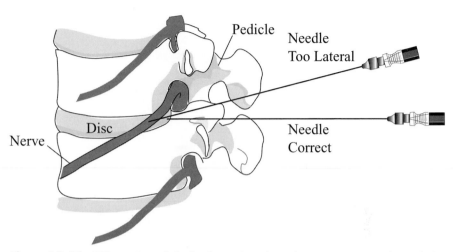

Figure 10–11. Oblique view of the lumbar spine where the nerve root exits beneath the pedicle and courses inferiorly and anteriorly. The discography needle should be placed just behind and below the nerve root to avoid neural injury. (From Zimmerman RA, Gibby WA, Carmody RF: Neuroimaging: Clinical and Physical Principles. New York, Springer-Verlag, Inc., 2000, p. 1443.)

the L5-S1 level to assess the height of the iliac crest and the size of the transverse processes.

   c. Hints to improve the chances of proper L5-S1 placement include:

     (1) Moving slightly more medial (the iliac crest tends to be higher more laterally)

     (2) Starting slightly higher than the level of the disc and angling inferiorly

     (3) Making sure an adequate number of rolled towels are underneath the patient to help rotate the iliac crest out of the way

     (4) The curved cannula that is provided in the nucleotome kit can be utilized. The disadvantage to the cannula is that it is somewhat larger in order to accommodate the curving of the nucleotome. The curved cannula can also be somewhat difficult to position.

C. Dilator

   1. The inner dilator and cannula are advanced over the flex trocar.

   2. The inner dilator is removed.

   3. The outer cannula is advanced 1–2 mm to ensure that the dilator is firmly against the annulus.

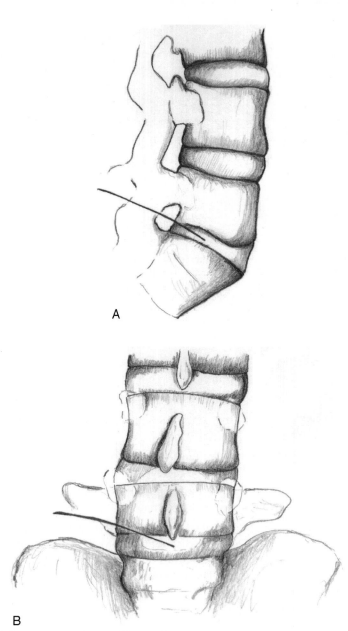

Figure 10–12. *A*, Lateral projection showing the needle correctly positioned in the central to posterior aspect of the disc. *B*, AP projection with the needle centrally located in the disc.

4. A gentle tap on the dilator can be used to assess for radicular pain, especially if the instrument is close to the nerve root.

D. Cutting device: A small cutting device is inserted and slowly turned with pressure, creating a fenestration in the annulus.

E. Nucleotome insertion: With one hand kept firmly on the cannula while holding it against the annulus, the inner cutter is removed and the probe is inserted (Fig. 10–13).

F. Disc Removal

1. The ridge on the percutaneous probe correlates with the cutting port of the cannula.

2. The operator should begin aspirating with the port closest to the herniation.

3. With one hand always kept on the outer cannula, the percutaneous probe is moved in and out of the disc and the entire unit is angled in different directions to aspirate as much of the nucleus as possible.

4. A black line on the nucleotome indicates when the port has been pulled inside of the cannula. Withdrawing the device beyond this is not wise because one may lose the position of the device within the disc and even potentially aspirate structures outside of the disc.

5. Toward the end of the procedure, ask the patient to alternately flex and extend the spine in order to push more disc toward the nucleotome.

6. Flushing of the disc with sterile saline followed by aspiration can increase disc removal yield.

7. Disc material is aspirated until no further material is retrieved (usually about 20–25 minutes).

8. On average, 3–5 g of disc material is removed.

9. In most cases, the total procedure time including the pre-procedure discography is about 45 to 90 minutes, depending on the difficulty of trocar placement.

VIII. Post-procedure Care

A. The patient is kept approximately 6 hours for observation and discharged.

B. Follow-up by phone is made the following day, and the patient is re-examined at one week.

C. Medications

1. 30 mg of Toradol is given intramuscularly to limit paraspinous muscle spasms.

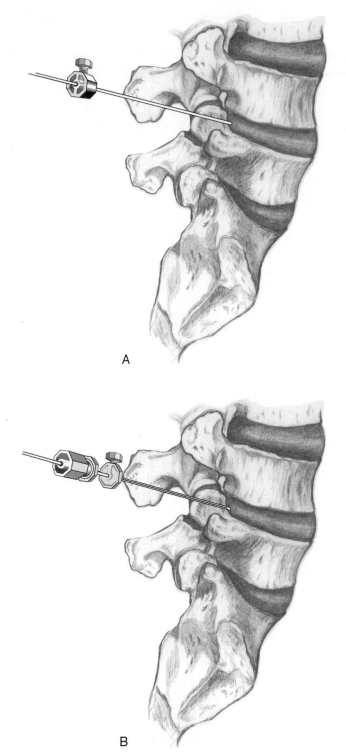

Figure 10–13. Percutaneous discectomy steps. *A*, Trocar inserted into disc. *B*, Dilator inserted followed by cutting cannula.

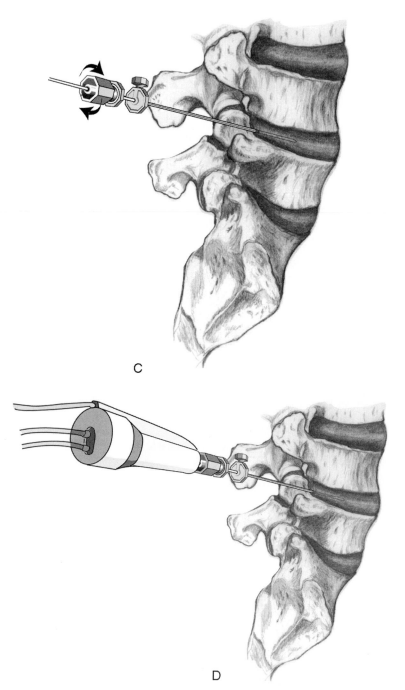

C

D

Figure 10–13 *Continued. C*, Annulus is fenestrated with the cutting cannula. *D*, Percutaneous probe is inserted. (From Zimmerman RA, Gibby WA, Carmody RF: Neuroimaging: Clinical and Physical Principles. New York, Springer-Verlag, Inc., 2000, p. 1492.)

2. I limit the patient's access to post-procedure narcotics to a single prescription.
3. In some patients muscle relaxants are also prescribed.

IX. Procedure Reporting

A. A history and physical examination are placed in the patient's chart prior to the procedure as per hospital policy.
B. The discography report is dictated separately from the percutaneous discectomy report.
C. SOAP (subjective, objective, assessment, and plan) notes are written on the patient's chart prior to discharge.
D. Brief follow-up notes are also transmitted to referring physicians. It is vital for the radiologists performing this procedure to take responsibility for their patients, including complications.

X. Procedural Coding

	CPT Code
A. Discography CPT Codes	
1. Discography—Lumbar	72295
2. Injection Procedure, Lumbar Discography	62290
3. Discography—Cervical or Thoracic	72285
4. Injection Procedure, Cervical or Thoracic Discography	62291
B. Percutaneous Discectomy Codes	
1. Percutaneous Discectomy—Lumbar	62287
2. Additional Lumbar Percutaneous Discectomy	62290
3. Percutaneous Discectomy—Cervical or Thoracic	62291
4. Fluoroscopy Charge—Up to 1 Hour	76000
5. Fluoroscopy Charge—Greater than 1 hour	76001

SUGGESTED READING

1. Mixter WJ, Barr JS: Rupture of the intervertebral disc with involvement of the spinal cord. N Engl J Med 211:210–214, 1934.
2. Bernard TN: Repeat lumbar spine surgery: factors influencing outcome. Spine 18(15):2196–2200, 1993.
3. Abramovitz JN: Complications of surgery for discogenic disease of the spine. Neurosurg Clin N Am 4:167–176, 1993.

4. Deyo RA, Loeser JD, Bigos SJ: Herniated lumbar intervertebral disk. Ann Intern Med 112:598–603, 1990.
5. Markwalder Th.-M, Battaglia M: Failed back surgery syndrome. Part I. Analysis of the clinical presentation and results of testing procedures for instability of the lumbar spine in 171 patients. Acta Neurochir 123:46–51, 1993.
6. Onik G, Helms C, Ginsburg L, et al: Percutaneous lumbar discectomy using a new aspiration probe. AJNR 6:290–293, 1985.
7. Onik G, Marron J, Helms C, et al: Automated percutaneous discectomy: initial patient experience. Radiology 162:129–132, 1987.
8. Maroon JC, Onik G, Sternau L: Percutaneous automated discectomy: a new approach to lumbar surgery. Clin Orthop 238(1):64–70, 1989.
9. Goldstein TB, Mink JH, Dawson EG: Early experience with automated percutaneous lumbar discectomy in the treatment of lumbar disc herniation. Clin Orthop 238(1):77–82, 1989.
10. Frank EH: Percutaneous discectomy—update. Epitomes Neurosurg 162(3):257–258, 1995.
11. Romy M: Percutaneous discectomy: an update. Semin Ultrasound CT MR 14(6):455–457, 1993.
12. Davis GW, Onik G. Clinical experience with automated percutaneous lumbar discectomy. Clin Orthop 238:98–103, 1989.
13. Mayer HM: Spine update: percutaneous lumbar disc surgery. Spine 19(23):2719–2723, 1994.
14. Mirovsky Y, Neuwirth MG, Halperin N: Automated percutaneous discectomy for reherniations of lumbar discs. J Spinal Disord 7(2):181–184, 1994.
15. Ho PSP, Yu S, Sether LA, et al: Progressive and regressive changes in the nucleus pulposus. Part I. Neonate. Radiology 169:87–91, 1988.
16. Taylor TKF, Akeson WH: Intravertebral disc prolapse: a review of the morphologic and biochemic knowledge concerning the nature of prolapse. Clin Orthop 76:54–79, 1971.
17. Wiesel SW, Tsourmas N, Feffer HL, et al: A study of computer assisted tomography: I. The incidence of positive CAT scans in an asymptomatic group of patients. Spine 9:549–551, 1989.

11

Intradiscal Electrothermal Therapy

Timothy S. Eckel, M.D., M.S.

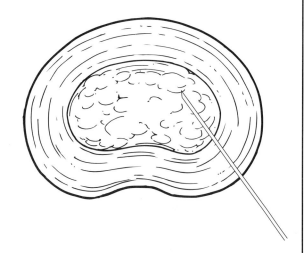

I. Rationale and Clinical Indications

A. Chronic low back pain is a common complaint, and management of low back pain is a formidable task for the spine specialist.

B. While poorly understood, the *discogenic* or *discopathic* pain mechanism has progressively gained acceptance as one source of chronic low back pain.

1. Discogenic pain is typically characterized by axial low back pain that is greater than leg pain, usually exacerbated by sitting or standing for prolonged periods of time.

2. Diagnosis of discogenic pain is based on classic clinical history (pain diagram) and pain-provocative discography with provocation of typical concordant pain symptoms on disc distention.

3. Theories for the exact pathophysiology of the pain mechanism abound, but most revolve around pathologic tears of the posterior annulus of the disc and mechanical or chemical stimulation of nociceptive fibers located in and around the posterior annulus fibrosus and relayed through the sinuvertebral nerve (Fig. 11–1).

C. Current therapy for discogenic pain includes continuation of conservative pain management regimens or surgery.

1. Conservative measures include rest, physical therapy, anti-inflammatory agents and analgesics, epidural steroids, chiropractic, and acupuncture, for example. Patients have generally not been helped by a 6-month course of conservative therapy prior to consideration for intradiscal electrothermal therapy (IDET).

2. Surgical intervention typically consists of discectomy and interbody fusion, which has yielded mixed results in treating discogenic pain; it may have significant complications and is considerably more costly than IDET.

D. IDET is a minimally invasive therapy for chronic discogenic low back pain refractory to conservative measures.

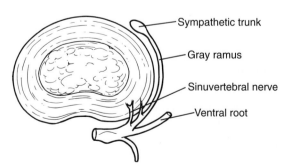

Figure 11–1. Innervation of the disc annulus.

1. IDET is a novel method of management for discogenic pain using intradiscal delivery of thermal energy to the internal structure of the disc annulus. Delivery of thermal energy is a common technique used for both pain management and tissue ablation, and has been shown to

   a. Shrink and reorient collagen fibrils

   b. Coagulate nerve tissue

   c. Cauterize granulation tissue

2. Extensive in vivo studies have demonstrated the IDET method to be a safe technique for applying thermal energy to the disc annulus for the purpose of shrinking disc substance, promoting annular healing and granulation, and coagulating nerve tissue in the annulus to treat discogenic pain.

3. Technical aspects of the procedure were developed in the mid-1990s. The first case was performed in 1997 under institutional review board approval. FDA approval was given in 1998.

E. Clinical indications: IDET is useful in treating chronic, activity-limiting discogenic low back pain that has been refractory to conservative measures.

1. Function-limiting low back pain of at least 6 months' duration

2. Back pain greater than leg pain with no true radicular symptoms

3. Failure to improve significantly with a comprehensive nonoperative back care program, including

   a. Progressive exercise (physical therapy)

   b. At least one fluoroscopic epidural injection

   c. A course of anti-inflammatory medication

   d. Activity modification

4. Magnetic resonance imaging (MRI) with no extruded disc fragments and no neural impingement

5. Pain-provocative discogram with concordant pain reproduction on low pressure injection at one or more disc levels

F. Results

1. Results are fairly consistent in many presentations and a few publications, although published data in peer-reviewed journals are sparse, and no placebo or sham trial exists at present.

2. Multiple citations report quite similar results, including several retrospective multicenter analyses, a few published prospective clinical trials, and a case-control study that compared procedural outcome with outcome in nontreated patients denied insurance coverage.

3. All trials generally reported a roughly 70%–75% response rate mea-

sured as a decrease in subjective pain on a visual analogue scale (VAS) with measurable decrease in analgesic use and measurable functional improvement (SF-36 scales) measured at 3, 6, and 12 months after the procedure.

II. Contraindications

A. Nerve root compression (radicular pain distribution or motor findings on examination)

B. Extruded disc fragment

C. Active infection and/or discitis

D. Bleeding disorder

E. Severe degenerative disc disease with >50% decrease in disc height; this is a relative contraindication that may preclude catheter navigation or placement within the disc.

III. Informed Consent

A. IDET is very safe if performed carefully by a skilled operator, and complications are very rare (≤2% in our experience). Risks are generally those associated with any needle puncture, plus the additional potential risks of traversing nerve damage on disc access, disc herniation from catheter manipulation, and localized nerve damage from thermal energy application.

B. Informed consent paperwork should include the following risks:

1. Allergy to local anesthetics or sedatives used

2. Bleeding

3. Infection

4. Nerve damage

5. Disc herniation (theoretical risk)

6. Risks associated with sedatives

C. Discussion with the patient should also touch on the uncertain long-term results (beyond 3 years) for this recently developed procedure.

IV. Pertinent Anatomy

A. Lumbar vertebra and radiographic appearance (Fig. 11–2)

1. Body and endplates

2. Pedicle

3. Articular processes

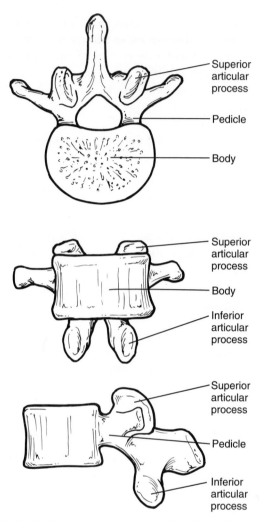

Figure 11–2. Vertebral anatomy (superior-inferior, AP, and lateral projections).

B. Lumbar disc (Fig. 11–3)

    1. Nucleus pulposus: Introducer needle position should be in nucleus.

    2. Annulus fibrosus

        a. Annular tears are related to pain production and discogenic pain.

        b. Annular tears allow ingrowth of vasculature and nociceptive pain fibers.

        c. Optimal catheter position results in heating element draped across entire posterior annulus.

C. Spinal nerve

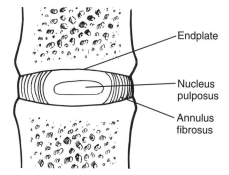

Figure 11–3. Intervertebral disc anatomy.

1. The course of the descending lumbar nerve root from the level above the disc to be treated descends obliquely across the lateral aspect of the disc.
2. Disc access is chosen to allow positioning of the introducer needle in the nucleus of the disc while avoiding the descending root (Fig. 11–4).

V. Equipment Requirements

A. Multidirectional fluoroscopy
B. 10-ml syringe for local anesthetic
C. 1.5-inch, 25 gauge infiltrating needle for skin anesthesia
D. 3.5-inch, 22 gauge spinal needle (deep anesthesia)

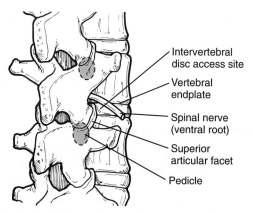

Figure 11–4. Right posterior oblique projection demonstrating the course of the spinal nerve across the disc. The safe entry zone for access to the disc is outlined by the roughly triangular region defined by the superior articular facet posteriorly, the superior endplate of the vertebral body inferiorly, and the spinal nerve medially and above.

E. 17-gauge introducer needle

F. SpineCATH catheter

G. ElectroThermal Spine System Generator

H. Connecting wires

I. Medications

　1. Local anesthetic (1% lidocaine or 0.25% bupivacaine)

　2. Antibiotics (e.g., cefazolin, 1 g)

VI. Sedation

A. Conscious sedation (neuroleptanalgesia) is typically with midazolam and fentanyl given intravenously.

　1. Midazolam is titrated slowly to effect a drowsy but rousable state; the patient should not be oversedated and must remain responsive during the procedure to report nerve root irritation symptoms if a root is encountered during disc access or during catheter manipulation.

　2. Fentanyl is slowly titrated to relieve pain provoked during application of thermal energy in the disc. (*Caution*: Fentanyl should be used only to reduce typical discogenic pain during heating and not to mask leg pain or radicular symptoms that may indicate improper position of the heating element with potential nerve damage.)

　3. Sedation requires nursing support/supervision with continuous monitoring of cardiac rhythm and pulse oximetry and intermittent automatic blood pressure monitor.

B. Local anesthesia: lidocaine or bupivacaine

VII. Procedure

A. Following informed consent, the patient is placed prone on the fluoroscopy table, and midazolam sedation is initiated while the low back is prepared and draped. The preparation area should be approximately equivalent to that used for discography.

B. The disc to be treated is visualized fluoroscopically, and the fluoroscope is angled parallel to the disc, flattening endplates above and below (typically craniocaudal angulation for L4-L5 and L5-S1 disc levels, and caudocranial angulation for L1-L2 and L2-L3 levels) (Fig. 11–5).

C. Fluoroscope is obliqued laterally to visualize and select the appropriate site of disc entry.

　1. The site of entry is chosen to allow access to the anterior aspect of

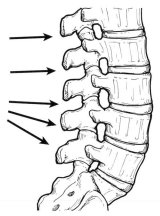

Figure 11–5. Lateral projection of the lumbar spine demonstrates angulation of the fluoroscope along the disc plane to facilitate visualization and disc access. Caudocranial angulation is required in the upper lumbar levels, and craniocaudal angulation is needed for the lower lumbar levels.

the disc nucleus while minimizing the chance of encountering the descending nerve root from the level above.

2. Appropriate obliquity is generally achieved when the superior articular facet has traversed between one third and one half of the disc (see Fig. 11–4).

3. In the oblique position, a triangular window for disc access is then defined by the superior facet medially, the superior endplate inferiorly, and the descending nerve root laterally and superiorly (see Fig. 11–4).

D. The skin is marked over the triangular disc access site with a radioopaque instrument or clamp, and local anesthesia is achieved with 2 ml of 1% lidocaine.

1. Local anesthesia is then carried down to the peridiscal soft tissues with a 3.5-inch spinal needle. The spinal needle is advanced slowly to avoid anesthetizing the descending nerve root crossing the disc. If the nerve is encountered, its position is noted, and the spinal needle is withdrawn and reoriented to approach the disc medially and below the position of the nerve root.

2. The stylet is replaced, and the spinal needle is withdrawn.

E. The 17-gauge introducer needle is then advanced along the trajectory of the spinal needle and into the disc. The needle is advanced slowly to avoid encountering the traversing root, and if radicular symptoms are elicited, the needle is withdrawn and reoriented to avoid the root.

1. A tactile resistance and gritty crunching are encountered when the

needle enters the annulus, and the fluoroscope is then repositioned in an anteroposterior (AP) projection.

2. Care should be taken not to advance the needle beyond the disc margins, and if there is any confusion about the position of the needle tip during advancement, its position should be checked in two orthogonal planes fluoroscopically.

3. The patient may report transient localized back pain as the needle penetrates the annulus. Radicular symptoms are not expected and may indicate needle position that is too close to the descending root.

F. Position is checked in the AP projection confirming position of the needle tip just inside the annulus, and the fluoroscope is rotated to the lateral projection.

G. The introducer needle is then advanced minimally to achieve positioning of the tip in the nucleus pulposus just in the anterior half of the disc. Optimal positioning occurs with the tip between 12 o'clock and 3 o'clock on a clock face (Fig. 11–6).

H. The SpineCATH catheter (Oratec Interventions, Menlo Park, CA) is then withdrawn from its sterile packaging. If desired, the catheter may be attached to the generator with the connecting wire to establish integrity of the system.

I. The needle is rotated to ensure that the opening in the needle tip points medially to facilitate catheter navigation. The stylet is removed from the introducer needle, and the catheter is advanced slowly into the needle until the distal marker on the catheter enters the needle hub, indicating that the catheter tip is about to exit the tip of the needle. The catheter must be aligned so that the curve in the catheter tip points medially to allow the curve in the catheter tip to deflect off the inner margin of the disc annulus.

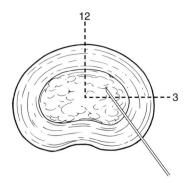

Figure 11–6. Axial projection demonstrating optimal introducer needle placement in the disc. Placement with tip just in the anterior half of the nucleus with the bevel open medially facilitates maneuvering the catheter along the inner margin of the annulus.

J. Under lateral fluoroscopy, the catheter is slowly advanced into the disc. Although a small amount of resistance is normal when the catheter first enters the disc, care should be taken that the catheter tip always advances when the proximal end is advanced to avoid binding the catheter tip on annular tears. The curve in the catheter is used to steer the catheter around the inner margin of the annulus.

  1. Lateral fluoroscopic monitoring allows the operator to visualize the catheter curving off the anterior and posterior margins of the annulus and to ensure that the catheter does not breach the anterior or posterior margins of the disc and enter either the retroperitoneum or the spinal canal. The catheter should be visualized gently curving off the anterior and posterior margins of the disc (Fig. 11–7) without extending significantly beyond the margins of the vertebral bodies above and below.

  2. Once the posterior curve is visualized and the catheter tip is no longer pointing directly posterior, the fluoroscope is reoriented in the AP projection.

  3. Catheter navigation can be performed either incrementally or with slow and gentle continuous pressure. Care must be taken to avoid binding the catheter in annular tears: if pressure is continually applied when the catheter tip is bound, the catheter may either rupture the annulus or kink within the disc. If resistance is met on advancing the catheter and the tip appears bound under fluoroscopy, two techniques may be helpful in catheter navigation.

     a. Catheter manipulation: The catheter can be partially withdrawn and turned to reorient the curved catheter tip in another direction (e.g., superior or inferior) to avoid the annular tear.

     b. Introducer needle manipulation: The opening in the introducer needle can be turned in a different direction to guide the catheter along another path, or the needle tip may be partially advanced or withdrawn to seek another path as long as the opening in the bevel remains within the nucleus.

     c. *Caution*: The catheter should be withdrawn so that it is entirely inside the needle prior to maneuvering the needle to eliminate the possibility of damaging or shearing the catheter.

  4. If the catheter becomes inadvertently kinked and is difficult to withdraw, the introducer needle should be partially withdrawn a few centimeters, and further attempts at removing the catheter can be made.

     a. If the catheter is not easily removed from the introducer and becomes bound to the needle tip, the catheter and needle should be gripped firmly together and withdrawn as a unit to avoid shearing the catheter.

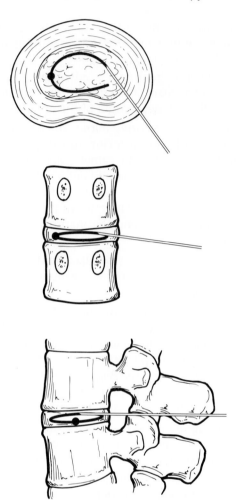

Figure 11-7. Axial, AP, and lateral projections demonstrating proper catheter positioning within the disc. The catheter should be positioned along the inner margin of the annulus fibrosus with the heating element of the catheter tip draped across annular tears and across the entire posterior margin of the annulus.

     b. The catheter should never be advanced or withdrawn forcefully when meeting resistance to avoid damage to the catheter and the possibility of shearing.

     c. A damaged catheter should never be heated, and it should be replaced.

  5. Catheter navigation is generally not painful for the patient, but it may rarely provoke some minor typical local back pain. If severe discomfort or radicular symptoms are encountered, manipulation

should be stopped and positioning should be carefully checked fluoroscopically to confirm catheter position within the disc.

K. The catheter is then slowly advanced to achieve positioning with the heating element (distal 2 inches of catheter from tip to radiopaque 2-inch marker) draped across the entire posterior annulus of the disc (pedicle to pedicle on the AP projection). The catheter position is examined and photographed in two projections to display:

1. Proper catheter position across the entire posterior annulus (see Fig. 11–7)

2. Positioning of the entire heating element outside the introducer needle

3. Positioning of the catheter so that no portion of the heating section is in contact with the introducer needle

L. *Note*: In extremely degenerated or desiccated discs, it may not be possible to navigate the entire posterior annulus without binding annular fissures. Every attempt at optimal positioning should be made, maneuvering the curved catheter tip and introducer as mentioned previously. If the catheter tip cannot be advanced beyond the midline of the posterior annulus, an initial treatment is carried out at the best achievable position, and the procedure should be repeated from the contralateral approach so that the entire posterior annulus is heated.

M. When proper positioning has been achieved, catheter positioning is documented in the AP and lateral planes.

1. If the heating element of the catheter projects over the introducer needle on the AP projection, an additional AP view with craniocaudal angulation is taken to document that the catheter heating element does not come into contact with the introducer needle.

2. The catheter is attached to the generator box with the sterile cable. The cable connection and the catheter are marked with white lines which are aligned directly, and the connectors snap together. No grounding cable is required, as the heating mechanism is resistive within the terminal 5 cm of the catheter.

N. The generator box is turned on. The resistance window should read about 120–280 in an intact catheter. If the reading is significantly higher than 280, the catheter may be damaged. It should be removed and replaced.

O. Once the equipment is appropriately attached, thermal energy is delivered with either a preset delivery program or with incremental heat increases controlled by hand.

1. Ideally, the catheter should be heated to 90°C for 4–6 minutes to deliver adequate energy to the annulus. The preset program in the

Oratec generator begins at 65°C and increases the temperature 1°C every 30 seconds until the 90°C level is reached.

2. A gradual increase in temperature is better tolerated than rapid temperature increases, although the increase can be varied according to the wishes of the treating physician.

P. The patient may report provocation of typical back pain and some typical referred pain with energy delivery, which can be controlled with intravenous analgesics at the discretion of the treating physician. True radicular symptoms should not be encountered, however, and if pain radiating to the leg is reported, energy delivery should be halted at once by pressing the RF power button on the generator, and the catheter should be repositioned.

Q. After treatment, the catheter is withdrawn with a steady pull, with care taken to avoid snagging the catheter on the introducer needle.

1. Intradiscal antibiotics may be injected at the discretion of the treating physician as a prophylaxis against potential disc infection. The needle track is anesthetized with local anesthetic as the introducer needle is withdrawn.

2. *Note:* If catheter position was suboptimal and a second treatment from the contralateral approach is required, no antibiotics should be injected until the second treatment is complete.

R. Hemostasis is achieved with a few minutes of manual compression, and the entry site is dressed with a sterile bandage.

S. The patient is discharged home with a caretaker after appropriate recovery from the analgesia with instructions not to drive.

T. Discharge instructions should include bed rest with no strenuous physical activity for 1–3 days.

U. Pearls

1. L5-S1 access may be difficult, and close correlation should be made with the pre-procedural discogram.

   a. For a low L5-S1 disc, placing a pillow or bolster under the patient's abdomen flattens the lumbar lordosis and increases accessibility to the low disc.

   b. For experienced practitioners, the 17-gauge introducer needle may be bent carefully on a needle bender to allow access. (The needle should be bent in such a manner so that the opening in the bevel will point medially after access.)

2. If the discogram demonstrated a lateralizing annular tear, needle approach is typically selected from the opposite side so that the heating element of the catheter will be draped across the annular tear.

VIII. Post-procedure Care

A. Efficacy of the procedure depends not only on its technical aspects but also on strict post-procedural guidelines that allow healing within the disc and avoidance of reinjury. Many practitioners give a printed instruction sheet with "do's and don'ts" and exercise instructions to patients after treatment.

B. Many patients experience an increase in typical symptoms for 1–7 days after the procedure with transient local discomfort at the entry site(s). Pain can be managed with local ice at the injection site and nonsteroidal anti-inflammatory drugs (NSAIDs) as needed. Patients with more severe pain or patients accustomed to narcotics may require narcotic analgesics as well. Most patients return to their pre-procedure pain level within the first week.

   1. Many practitioners recommend a fitted lumbar corset to be worn during waking hours for the first few weeks after the procedure.

   2. The patient should be instructed to call if fever develops or if post-procedural flareup does not resolve after the first week.

C. Symptomatic improvement usually begins 1–2 weeks after treatment, and symptoms continue to improve gradually over time for as long as 6–9 months.

D. Pain control

   1. Symptoms can usually be managed with local ice, rest, mild activity restrictions, and NSAIDs.

   2. Moderately severe pain may be managed additionally with a lumbar corset and potentially with narcotic analgesics.

   3. Severe pain may require significant activity restrictions (1–2 days of bed rest) with NSAIDs and narcotic analgesics. Some consideration may be given to a bolus and rapid taper of oral steroids or epidural steroids, although care must be taken to ensure that there is no infection (consider white blood cell count with differential and erythrocyte sedimentation rates).

E. Restrictions

   1. Rest 1–3 days after procedure.

   2. Avoid prolonged vertical sitting: Limit to 30–40 minutes for the first 2 weeks, then increase as tolerated.

   3. No heavy lifting or strenuous upper-body activity. Lifting restrictions: 1–10 lb for first 2 weeks, then 25–50 lb for first 3 months

   4. Avoid twisting and forward bending.

   5. Corset (optional) should be worn for 2 weeks, and then as needed for comfort or pain flareups.

F. Exercise and activity

1. Return to work time varies for the individual patient and type of work. Most patients can return to sedentary work 2–5 days after the procedure, although they should be instructed not to sit in one position for more than 30–40 minutes at a time. Patients should not return to heavy work or lifting before week 8 and should engage in some individualized and progressive work hardening before return to work.

2. Light housework may resume at 1 week.

3. In week 2, patients should be encouraged to begin exercise with walking only, and to begin stretching exercises. Walking and stretching are encouraged for the remainder of the recovery period to maintain flexibility and promote healing.

4. Exercise should include walking beginning at week 2 and may progress as tolerated to include stationary bicycling and swimming (no flip turns). Jarring axial loads (Use of a Stairmaster, running, rowing, aerobics) should be avoided.

5. Daily stretching exercises are encouraged. Abdominal and back-strengthening exercises are encouraged (knee to chest, and pelvic brace). More strenuous exercises are added as tolerated after week 4 (bridging, abdominal curls).

6. Patients who are slow to recover or need more detailed instructions may be referred for a formal physical therapy program for back stabilization at 6 weeks if they are tolerating advancing activity.

7. Weightlifting may resume in month 3. Axial loads are to be avoided (no back or abdominal machines, no torso twisting, no overhead lifts or squats).

8. Athletic pursuits can be resumed in month 4 depending on tolerance of increased activity. Golf and tennis may require special instruction.

IX. Procedure Reporting

A. Rationale (discogenic pain)

B. Informed consent

C. Level(s) treated

D. Approach (unilateral or bilateral): Comment on catheter positioning (i.e., optimal, pedicle to pedicle, or suboptimal requiring bilateral treatment)

E. Medications administered (sedation and intradiscal if given)

F. Equipment (e.g., Oratec generator)

G. Time of catheter heating for each application

1. Standard treatment protocol is for a total of 16.5 minutes to a maximum of 90°C for 6 minutes.

2. Describe any symptoms elicited on catheter heating.

H. Disposition: Include discussion of expectations for the patient regarding post-procedure care and exercise and therapy regimen.

X. Procedural Coding

A. Dependent on locality and local rules and regulations

B. Pre-certification is suggested, because the procedure is not uniformly covered by insurance carriers at date of press.

C. Possible physician codes to consider

	CPT Code
1. Aspiration or decompression procedure, percutaneous, of nucleus pulposus of intervertebral disc, any method, single or multiple levels, lumbar	62287
2. Destruction by neurolytic agent, chemical, thermal, electrical of peripheral nerve or branch	64640
3. Fluoroscopic guidance and localization of needle or catheter tip for spine or paraspinous diagnostic or therapeutic injection procedure	76005-26
4. Discography, lumbar, radiologic supervision and interpretation	72295
5. Sedation with or without analgesia (conscious sedation), intravenous, intramuscular, or inhalation	99141
6. Unlisted procedure, nervous system	64999
7. Unlisted procedure, spine	22899

SUGGESTED READING

1. Derby R, Eek B, Chen Y, et al: Intradiscal electrothermal annuloplasty (IDET): a novel approach for treating chronic low back pain. Neuromodulation 3(2):82–88, 2000.
2. Elias WJ, Simmons NE, Kaptain GJ, et al: Complications of posterior lumbar interbody fusion when using a titanium threaded cage device. J Neurosurg 93(Suppl 1):45–52, 2000.
3. Freemont AJ, Peacock TE, Goupille P, et al: Nerve ingrowth into diseased intervertebral disc in chronic back pain. Lancet 350:178–181, 1997.
4. Hacker RJ: Comparison of interbody fusion approaches for disabling low back pain. Spine 22:660–665, 1997.
5. Karasek M, Bogduk N: Twelve-month follow-up of a controlled trial of intradiscal thermal annuloplasty for back pain due to internal disc disruption. Spine 25:2601–2607, 2000.
6. O'Neil C, Derby R, Kenderes L: Precision injection techniques for diagnosis and treatment of lumbar disc disease. Semin Spine Surg 11:104–118, 1999.
7. Ohtori S, Takahashi Y, Takahashi K, et al: Sensory innervation of the dorsal portion of the lumbar intervertebral disc in rats. Spine 24:2295–2299, 1999.
8. Parker LM, Murrell SE, Boden SD, Horton WC: The outcome of posterolateral fusion in highly selected patients with discogenic low back pain. Spine 21:1909–1917, 1996.

9. Rhyne AL, Smith SE, Wood KE, Darden BV. Outcome of unoperated discogram-positive low back pain. Spine 20:1997–2001, 1995.
10. Saal JS, Saal JA: Intradiscal electrothermal treatment for chronic discogenic low back pain: a prospective outcome study with minimum 1-year follow-up. Spine 25:2622–2627, 2000.
11. Saal JS, Saal JA: Management of chronic discogenic low back pain with a thermal intradiscal catheter: a preliminary study. Spine 25(3):382–388, 2000.
12. Thompson KJ, Eckel TS: IDET Nationwide Registry preliminary results: twelve month follow-up on 211 patients. Presented at North American Spine Society, New Orleans, October 2000.
13. Tiusanen H, Seitsalo S, Osterman K, Soini J: Anterior interbody lumbar fusion in severe low back pain. Clin Orthop 324:153–163, 1996.
14. Tiusanen H, Hurri H, Seitsalo S, et al: Functional and clinical results after anterior interbody lumbar fusion. Eur Spine J 5:288–292, 1996.
15. Vamvanij V, Fredrickson BE, Thorpe JM, et al: Surgical treatment of internal disc disruption: an outcome study of four fusion techniques. J Spinal Disord 11:375–382, 1998.

Index

245